"Beloved, I wish above all things that thou mayest prosper and be in health, even as thy soul prospereth" **(III John 2).**

Your Total Health Handbook

• Body • Soul • Spirit •

By Marilyn Hickey

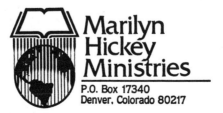

Marilyn Hickey Ministries

P.O. Box 17340
Denver, Colorado 80217

Your Total Health Handbook
• Body • Soul • Spirit •

Copyright © 1993 by Marilyn Hickey Ministries
P.O. Box 17340
Denver, Colorado 80217
All Rights Reserved
ISBN 1-56441-024-2

All scriptures are quoted from the *King James Version* of the Bible unless otherwise indicated.

Printed in the U.S.A.

CONTENTS

Section Four

Section Five

Section Six

Section Seven

Section Eight

Section Nine

Section Ten

Section Eleven

ENDNOTES

WORKS CITED

Section One
GUIDELINES FOR HEALTHY EATING

America ... world leader in medical and scientific technology ... the "promised land" ... flowing with milk and honey .... Yet millions of Americans are overweight, stricken with heart ailments, a multitude of cancers, and degenerative diseases. We spend billions of dollars on junk food, diet plans, and medical bills.

If you want to lose weight and/or gain health, you won't find your key to strength, vitality, and long life in the latest diet fad or processed, "convenience" frozen food. Your only key is a 4,000-year-old guide to life—the Bible. In His Word, God gave you all the information you need to have a healthy body, soul, and spirit. His plan for health is practical and profoundly simple.

This handy guidebook will aid you in studying God's Word as you strive to honor and glorify Him in all you do—the way you treat your body, control your emotions, and develop your spiritual walk (I Corinthians 10:31).

This guidebook will help you understand how the Mosaic laws for food (Leviticus 11) can help you eat better for life. I have searched the Scriptures and found God's principles to healthier eating through vegetables, fruit, meats, fish, bread, and more.

You will also learn how to shed the heavy weights of your heart—anger, worry, fear, anxiety, depression, and unforgiveness—so that when your body, heart, and mind are in line with God's Word, your spiritual walk will come even closer to Him.

EATING THE WRONG things led to the destruction of several people and their families in the Old Testament—Eli (I Samuel 4:11,18), Eglon (Judges 3:17-22), Esau (Genesis 25:29-34), and Adam and Eve (Genesis 3).

GOD GAVE DIETARY laws to the children of Israel before they went into the Promised land.

- The Canaanites ate anything (dogs, bugs, fat, blood), and

9

archeologists show that they suffered from heart disease, arthritis, cancer, and early death.

- God wanted His people to be prosperous and live long in the land He gave them.

SALVATION THROUGH CHRIST Jesus sets us free from living under the letter of the Mosaic law (Hebrews 10:1-10).

- God's guidelines for eating are being proven by medical and nutritional specialists to be the cheapest, easiest, and wisest way to live longer and with more strength, vitality, and health.

DANIEL AND HIS three friends became healthier and ten times wiser by refusing King Nebuchadnezzar's rich foods in order to obey God's dietary laws (Daniel 1:8-20).

- Daniel, Shadrach, Meshach, and Abednego ate *pulse* (vegetables, seeds, grains, and herbs) and water.

GOD CREATED PURE food to give you life; repair and build your muscles, organs, skin, hair, nails, blood, and bones; regulate your body temperature; give you strength, stamina, and vitality; and keep you fit.[1]

- God's ways are good, natural, balanced, and cannot be improved (Genesis 1:31).

LIVE CLOSE TO God. Even in this polluted world, try to live as close to God's sweet nature as possible.

- Try to stay out of polluted areas so you can breathe fresh air.
- Drink pure water, eat healthful foods, and communicate with your Lord through prayer and reading His Word.

NOT ALL THE foods available today are mentioned in the Bible because travel and communication were limited in Bible times and the Middle Eastern climate and geography restricted the type of crops grown.

- Eating all the varieties of vegetables and fruit in their natural state are as close as your diet can come to God's plan.
- Eat only fresh vegetables and fruit, not canned, frozen, or processed in any way. Eat them raw, lightly steamed, baked or stewed.

- Eat whole grains, nuts, and seeds.
- Eat fish and lean beef, lamb, chicken, and turkey.
- Include dairy foods—milk, cottage cheese, cheese, and yogurt—in your diet.[2]
- When you eat natural foods and do it to God's glory and honor, you will not go hungry and you will receive everything your body needs (I Corinthians 10:31; Proverbs 10:3).

PROCESSED, UNNATURAL FOODS do not add, and in some cases deplete, the nutrients your body needs to function. These canned, boxed, and packaged meals have had their enzymes, vitamins, and minerals stripped away.

- Processed foods are filled with toxins (preservatives, artificial flavors and colors, and synthetic vitamins) that your body doesn't need and will cause it damage.
- These foods may look and sometimes taste better than natural foods, but they will make your body heavy and sickly, and make you look older, feel horrible, and die young.[3]
- You can't remain healthy on a diet that is low in amino acids—which are the building blocks of protein, hormones, enzymes, and nucleic acids. Nucleic acids make up your genetic code, which is found in your DNA (deoxyribonucleic acid) and RNA (ribonucleic acid).
- The life of all flesh is in the blood (Leviticus 17:14). If the body is toxic with junk food and chemicals, the blood delivers poison to every cell.[4]

TO LOSE WEIGHT and remain healthy you must eat healthful foods, exercise, change your behavior and way of living, and raise your expectations of what you can accomplish with God's help (Isaiah 55:2).

- Change your diet for LIFE, not for a couple of weeks.[5]

EFFECTIVE WEIGHT LOSS and maintenance for almost anyone (excepting people who do heavy labor, such as lumberjacks and construction workers, and need a high caloric intake to meet their bodies' needs) can be achieved by eating 1,000 to 1,800 calories a day.

- Eat 50 percent vegetables, 25 percent whole grains, nuts, and seeds, and 25 percent dairy foods, meat, and fish.[6]
- Take in daily allowances of each food classification, protein, vitamins, and minerals.
- You need anywhere between 35 to 50 grams of fiber a day.

ONE POUND OF body fat equals 3,500 calories.

- You must burn 3,500 calories through exercise in order to lose one pound.
- To lose one pound a week, eat 500 fewer calories than you will burn each day.
- To lose two pounds a week, eat 1,000 fewer calories than you burn each day.[7]
- Don't try to lose more than two pounds a week. Rapid weight loss can lead to painful gallstones (which require medical attention, chemical treatments, and even surgery).

YOU, YOUR EATING, AND YOUR BODY

FRUIT

APPLES, FIGS, GRAPES, and pomegranates were most frequently mentioned in the Bible, but virtually any fruit remains within the spirit of the Bible diet.

- Fruit is low in fat, high in fiber, and full of vitamins. In fact, the vitamin content in fruit effectively complements the minerals found in vegetables, grains, and meat.[8]

WARNING: EATING A diet of only fruit can be fatal!

- Americans have low amounts of copper in their diets (from eating too much overprocessed foods and vegetables and fruit grown in soil depleted of its minerals). This low level of copper mixed with a high dose of the sugar found in fruit, called fructose, can cause the heart to double in size, according to the U.S. Department of Agriculture.[9]

THE FOLLOWING ARE just some of the fruit you should eat daily.
- Eat different kinds every day to increase levels of different vitamins and minerals in your diet and to avoid boredom.
- Don't eat too much fruit. Your body doesn't need that much sugar, natural or not.

APPLES—Eat an apple or two a day to dampen your appetite and aid in weight control, and to keep the doctor bills at bay.
- Apples contain *chlorogenic acid*, which inhibits cancer in animals.
- Apples lower cholesterol and control blood pressure.
- They stabilize blood sugar, which is a bonus for diabetics or people prone to diabetes.[10]
  - 80 to 125 calories, depending on size
  - vitamins A, C, niacin, folate, other B vitamins
  - calcium, magnesium, potassium, phosphorous, iron[11]

MELONS—Cantaloupe, casaba, honeydew, and watermelon are excellent heart foods!
- Fiber and adenosine (an anti-coagulant also found in garlic and onions) in melons help dissolve the blood clots inside arteries that can cause heart attacks and strokes.
- Melon's high percentage of potassium helps lower and regulate blood pressure.
  - 45-55 calories per cup
  - vitamin A, beta carotene, vitamin C
  - potassium[12]

APRICOTS—Scientists say the Hunza people of the Himalaya Mountains have extraordinarily long and healthy lives because they eat a great quantity of apricots and yogurt and only a little meat.[13]
  - 17 calories per apricot
  - vitamin A, beta carotene, B vitamins
  - calcium, iron, copper, potassium[14]

FIGS—Isaiah used figs to treat King Hezekiah, who was "sick unto death." I believe he had skin cancer (Isaiah 38:1,21).
- A cancer-fighting chemical called benzaldehyde is abundant

in figs.

- The USDA says figs can curb your appetite.
- Enzymes in figs aid digestion.
- Fig juice can kill certain harmful bacteria.
  - 37 calories per medium raw fig; 46 calories per one dried fig
  - vitamins A, C
  - calcium, magnesium, potassium[15]

GRAPES—Mentioned most often in the Bible, grapes are capable of killing viruses, including polio and herpes simplex.

- Grape juice can kill bacteria and halt tooth decay.
- The caffeic acid in grapes may also help prevent cancer.
- Raisins, dried grapes, are as rich in the same vitamins and minerals as grapes but are easier to carry with you as an easy, "anytime" snack.
  - 58 calories per one cup grapes raw; 237 per ½ cup raisins
  - vitamins A, C, some B vitamins
  - calcium, potassium, zinc[16]

POMEGRANATES—The crimson pulp is filled with seeds that give a tasty burst of vitamin C.

- High in potassium, pomegranates can help control blood pressure.
  - 104 calories in a medium fruit
  - vitamin C, some B vitamins
  - potassium, calcium, iron[17]

BERRIES—Blackberries, blueberries, raspberries, and strawberries are rich in fructose and fiber, so they give a boost of energy along with vitamins and minerals!

- Raspberries and blackberries are rich in insoluble fiber, which is also found in whole grains. We need between 20 and 50 grams of insoluble fiber each day to regulate the digestive system and block calorie absorption.
- Berries have a lot of potassium, so they help control blood pressure.

- 45 to 80 calories per cup, depending on berry
- vitamin C[18]

CHERRIES—Eat cherries to satisfy your sweet tooth and prevent tooth decay!

- Atlanta's Forsyth Dental Center said results of their studies show cherry juice blocks nearly 90 percent of plaque formation by neutralizing enzyme activity.[19]
- Eat six to ten cherries daily to control or eliminate gout (an acute inflammation of the joints).[20]
- 80 calories raw per cup; 114 water packed
- vitamins A, C
- calcium, magnesium, potassium, iron[21]

CURRANTS—Get sugar-free currant jelly.

- Currants contain anti-bacterial chemicals that can keep blood vessels clear of cholesterol and fat-laden plaque deposits.
- 62 to 72 calories per cup
- vitamins A, C, some B vitamins
- calcium, potassium, magnesium, zinc, phosphorus, iron[22]

ORANGES—Oranges and other citrus fruit may lower cholesterol. Researchers at the University of South Florida say pectin fiber in citrus binds with cholesterol and whisks it out of the body before it can collect on artery walls.[23]

- 60 calories per medium orange; 110 calories per cup of unsweetened juice
- vitamins A, C, some B vitamins
- calcium, potassium, phosphorus[24]

VEGETABLES

VEGETABLES REDUCE FAT in your body, provide a high quantity of fiber to improve digestion, contain many essential minerals, are free of fat and sodium, and are low in calories.

GARLIC—This marvelous vegetable may be what helped prevent epidemics among the thousands of slaves in Egypt who lived in squalid, dirty conditions while expending so much energy to build Egyptian showpieces.

- Allicin in raw garlic fights germs and boosts the immune system.
- Cooked garlic can lower cholesterol, thin the blood, and act as a decongestant and cough medicine.
- Odorless garlic pills are especially good for cardiovascular benefits.[25]
  - 13 calories in 10 cloves
  - vitamin C
  - calcium, magnesium, potassium[26]

ONIONS, LEEKS—Onions have the same benefits as garlic!

- Eat an onion a day to raise your "good" HDL (high-density lipoprotein) cholesterol by 30 percent—as much or more than regular aerobic exercise.
- Onions promote better circulation and dissolve dangerous clots.
- They fight bacterial infections, bronchitis, and congestion; and may block cancer.[27]
  - 54 calories in a full onion
  - vitamin C, some B vitamins
  - potassium, calcium[28]

RADISHES—These small vegetables contain properties that kill a number of bacteria.

  - 7 calories in 10 radishes
  - vitamins A, C
  - calcium, magnesium, potassium, iron[29]

CUCUMBERS—The Israelites desperately missed and whined to Moses about one of their favorite foods, cucumbers, while in the desert (Numbers 11:5).

- Cucumbers are an excellent weight loss food.
- They promote easy digestion, cleanse the bowels, detoxify the system, and clear the skin.

- 32 calories per 8 oz[30]

CRUCIFEROUS VEGETABLES—The cabbage family is important because it provides some of the most important nutrients for health and long life.

- Cruciferous vegetables provide powerful cancer prevention, especially against colon and rectal cancers.
- The chemicals *indoles* and *dithiolithiones,* as well as beta carotene and vitamin C, are at work in these vegetables to prevent cancer in your body.
- Cruciferous vegetables are filled with calcium, which may fight degenerative diseases and osteoporosis, a breakdown of the bone mass.
- Eat cruciferous vegetables on a daily basis to get all the health protection you need (but don't eat the same thing every day).
- When cooking these vegetables, boil or steam them. They retain most of their vitamins and minerals this way, and neither method adds unnecessary fat.

BROCCOLI—24 calories per raw cup, 46 per cooked
- vitamins A, C, some B vitamins
- calcium, potassium, magnesium, zinc, phosphorus

BRUSSELS SPROUTS—60 calories per cup cooked
- vitamin C, beta carotene
- calcium, magnesium, potassium, phosphorus, iron, zinc

CABBAGE—32 calories per cup cooked
- vitamin A
- calcium, potassium, zinc

CAULIFLOWER—30 calories per cup cooked
- vitamin C
- calcium, potassium, magnesium, phosphorus, zinc

KALE—42 calories per cup cooked
- vitamin A, C
- calcium, potassium, iron[31]

LEAFY GREEN VEGETABLES—Eat beet greens, chicory greens, collard greens, lettuce, mustard greens, spinach, Swiss chard, and turnip greens in salads or shred and add them to soups, casseroles, lasagna, stir-fries, and stuffings.

- Leafy greens are high in fiber, beta carotene, and vitamin C.[32]

RED, YELLOW, AND ORANGE VEGETABLES—Heaped abundantly in your supermarket, these versatile and tasty vegetables were not available during Bible times, but their goodness would have made them excellent candidates for inclusion in Bible diets.

- Red, yellow, and orange vegetables have a high content of beta carotene (which the liver converts into vitamin A) which is noted for preventing degenerative disease, including cancer.[33]

CARROTS—Considered a tremendous cancer fighter, studies show that eating one carrot every day can reduce your risk of lung cancer (if you don't smoke) by half.

- National Cancer Institute investigators found this anti-cancer effect also applies to malignancies of the pancreas, throat, colon, prostate, cervix, and bladder.
- Carrots have a high amount of beta carotene. The recommended daily allowance for beta carotene is 5,000 International Units (IU). Cancer investigators say 12,500 IU is needed to prevent cancer. Two and a half carrots have 39,000 IU!
- Carrots may also lower cholesterol and improve digestion.
  - 31 calories per raw; 70 per cup cooked
  - vitamin C, beta carotene
  - calcium, potassium, magnesium, phosphorus, iron[34]

STARCHY VEGETABLES—Scientists say starchy vegetables (legumes, tubers, and roots) protect you against heart disease and diabetes, improve your digestion, and block cancer formation.

- The children of Israel primarily ate bread, water, lentils, onions, and yams while doing all their forced labor (such as building pyramids).

- Legumes, such as peas and beans, have a great deal of soluble fiber and vegetable protein.
- Tubers and roots, such as potatoes and yams, give us energy with all of their complex carbohydrates, vitamins, minerals, fiber, and muscle-building protein.[35]

BEANS—Pinto, white, navy, great northern, black, fava, and kidney beans; and black-eyed peas and chickpeas are really a seed food and contain the vegetable protein that builds muscles.

- Nutritionists say you should eat beans with rice, potatoes, or pasta (strict starch foods) to get the complete protein found in meat, which contains amino acids necessary for health.[36]
- Beans bind with dangerous LDL (low-density lipoprotein) cholesterol and improve the ratio of "good" HDL cholesterol.
- Soluble fiber, plant gums, and pectin in beans bind with fatty, cholesterol-laden clusters in the digestive tract and speeds them out of the body.
- Beans regulate insulin and blood sugar levels by slowing the rise of blood sugar enough so the pancreas doesn't have to keep pumping out high amounts of insulin.[37]
- They reduce high blood pressure, lower cholesterol, and prevent heart attacks and angina.
- Beans prevent constipation, hemorrhoids, and other bowel disorders because there are 10-20 grams of dietary fiber in a one-cup serving of the average dried bean—the National Cancer Institute recommends a daily minimum of 25 to 30 grams of fiber.
- Beans contain protease inhibitors, chemicals which can block the cancer development process.[38]
- The body converts the bean compound, lignan, into hormones that can halt cancer growth in the breast and colon.
  - ■ 241 calories per cooked cup

19

- niacin, folic acid, other B vitamins
- calcium, potassium, iron, magnesium, zinc, phosphorus, copper[39]

LENTILS—Genesis 25:29-34 talks about Jacob's lentil pulse, called pottage, that tempted Esau into forfeiting his birthright. This same meal can be one of the most nutritious foods you can eat today—without losing anything but ill health.

- You can combine lentils with rice pilaf or add to soups, stews, salads, and casseroles. Mix lentils with onions, garlic, and grains to make lentil stew.
- A staple in the Middle East, lentils are an ideal protein food because they contain virtually no fat.
- A cup of cooked lentils delivers a gram more protein than three ounces of lean ground beef.
  - 231 calories per boiled cup
  - vitamins A, C, folate
  - calcium, magnesium, zinc, potassium, phosphorous, iron, copper[40]

YAMS—Like other Bible foods, yams lower the risk of cancer and reduce cholesterol.

- Their dark yellow or orange coloring comes from their high concentration of beta carotene and other carotenoid compounds.
- Yams may slow diseases of aging, such as heart disease and arthritis, with chemicals that neutralize free-radicals (harmful metabolic by-products of breathing oxygen, such as carbon dioxide, and exposure to ultraviolet radiation and junk food).
- Polyphenols, which are abundant in yams, have antioxidant powers to cancel out free-radicals, in much the same way vitamins A, C and E and selenium do.
  - 118 calories in one baked yam
  - vitamin C, beta carotene
  - calcium, potassium, iron[41]

POTATOES—A source of fiber, vitamin C, and potassium, potatoes are a great weapon in the war against cholesterol, high blood pressure, and strokes.[42]

- Potatoes have an ample amount of protease inhibitors, which neutralize carcinogens and some viruses.
- Potato skins provide *chlorogenic acid*, which prevents certain cellular mutations that can become cancerous tumors.
- Ten plain baked potatoes have as many calories as four ounces of steak. Keep the calories low by topping with herbs, Worcestershire sauce, and a dab of non-fat yogurt.
  - 145 calories per baked potato
  - vitamin C, niacin, other B vitamins
  - magnesium, zinc, potassium, iron[43]

GRAINS

AT LEAST 25 percent of one or two of your daily meals should be whole grains, which you can eat plain and in muffins or breads.[44]

- Eating corn, beans, and rice can reduce the risk of heart disease and cancers of the colon, breast, and prostate.

BARLEY—Add uncooked barley to soups and stews, or add cooked barley to salads. Use barley flour or flakes for baking.

- Get whole-grain barley in health food stores, instead of Scotch or pearled barley.
- Naturally low in fat and cholesterol, it is an excellent source of soluble fiber.[45]
- USDA studies show compounds in barley can lower blood cholesterol.
- Barley may contain cancer-blocking chemicals.
  - 300 calories in a half cup
  - vitamins B1, B2, niacin
  - calcium, potassium, phosphorus, iron[46]

WHEAT—This abundant grain makes pita, which is a fat-free, flat bread eaten in Bible times and the current Middle East, and will give you strength and endurance (Exodus 12:34).

- Whole wheat is an excellent source of B vitamins and Vitamin E, which combine with vitamins A and C from other dietary sources to protect against cancer, heart disease, and other disorders.
- It aids digestion and prevents constipation.
  - 400 calories in a cup of whole-wheat flour
  - calcium, potassium, phosphorus[47]

CORN—Insist on eating fresh corn on the cob, or use cornmeal to make biscuits and breads.

- Corn is high in fiber and rich in complex carbohydrates that supply energy.
- Compounds in corn may prevent cancer.
- Corn has a very high quality vegetable protein.
  - 178 calories per cooked cup
  - vitamins A, C, some B vitamins
  - calcium, phosphorus, iron[48]

OATS—This high-fiber food has been shown to combat heart disease, lower cholesterol, check diabetes, and control insulin and blood sugar metabolism.

- Oats have a laxative effect, helping to lower the risk of cancer in the colon or digestive tract, because they are rich in fiber.
- Eat a half cup of cooked oat bran or one cup of dry oatmeal (cooked) every day.
  - 110 calories per ounce
  - B vitamins
  - calcium, magnesium, zinc, potassium, phosphorus, iron[49]

RICE—When you buy rice, remember that there is a substantial difference between the types of grains available—brown rice is the best source of nutrition; converted rice is next; but white rice is not nourishing.

- The staple food of the Chinese and Indian cultures, rice was cultivated in ancient Egypt as well.[50]
- It has the positive attributes of most other plant foods, plus

a healthful blast of vegetable protein.
- Rice can lower blood pressure, prevent kidney stones, relieve psoriasis, and may also contain chemicals to prevent cancer.
  - 232 calories per cooked cup
  - vitamin E, some B vitamins
  - calcium, potassium, phosphorus, iron[51]

NUTS AND SEEDS—For a wonderful snack, buy nuts and seeds in the shell and hull them yourself for greater nutritional value (make sure it says "raw" on the label).
- Seeds are rich in protein and minerals, but not when they are roasted and salted. They have lost most of their nutrients and are more difficult to digest, which is especially true of peanut butter.[52]
- Don't eat more than an ounce of nuts or seeds daily because they are high in fat.
- Nuts promote a steady rise in blood sugar and insulin, making them good snacks for diabetics and people who are prone to diabetes.
- Animal experiments show that nuts provide chemicals, protease inhibitors among them, which can block cancer development. Peanuts, almonds, Brazil nuts, cashews, pignolas, walnuts, and others all demonstrate this cancer-inhibiting ability.
  - some B vitamins
  - magnesium[53]

BREAD

BREAD IS THE Bible's principle food, and it can be found all the way from Genesis to Revelation.
- Bread was considered sacred, a gift of God. It was always broken and shared, a symbol of life, friendship and covenant relationships.
- Sometimes bread and water are the only forms of nourishment the Bible mentions, suggesting humans can

live by bread alone (I Kings 19:6).

EZEKIEL'S BREAD, FOUND in Ezekiel 4:9, is made from a variety of grains, which nutritionists tell us delivers more food value and higher quality protein than breads made from a single grain.[54] (Recipe is in SECTION 10.)

WHEN JESUS USED an example of life to explain Who He is to mankind, He said in John 6:35, "... *I am the bread of life: He that cometh to me shall never hunger; He that believeth on me shall never thirst.*"

- After His death and resurrection, Jesus appeared to two men. He didn't tell them Who He was, but when they sat down to break bread with Him, they recognized Him (Luke 24:30,31). It was through the breaking of bread that they knew Jesus!
- Jesus tells us to take communion by breaking bread so we can discern His body.
- When we eat bread, Jesus wants us to have a revelation that He is the Life, the True Bread from our Father.

YOU AND FAT

ABSTAINING FROM FAT made good sense even in the days of Moses. The wealthy and privileged ate huge amounts of high-fat meals and suffered the same hardening of the arteries, heart attacks and strokes that we do today.[55]

- While your body needs some fat, the type of fat found in animal foods—saturated fat—is not necessary in abundance.
- Only 25 percent of your daily intake should be meats, fish, or dairy products.[56]

ONE GRAM OF FAT is equal to 9 calories!

- To calculate the percentage of calories in your diet that comes from fat, multiply the number of fat grams in a serving by nine, and divide that number by the number of total calories in a serving. The number you get is the percentage of calories that comes from fat.[57]

- To lose weight, no more than 10 percent of your daily intake of calories should be fat calories.

CHOLESTEROL INFORMATION ABOUNDS and we are continually warned to steer clear of milk, eggs, butter, and meat—all of which are God-given, nutritious, healthful foods.

- Only one out of every 500 people needs to cut ALL animal fat out of his diet due to an inherited condition of super-high cholesterol called hypercholesterolemia.[58]
- When so-called authorities deprive us of necessary, life-giving foods, they are violating Biblical principles (Genesis 9:4; Leviticus 11; I Kings 4:23; Isaiah 7:15; Acts 27:34; I Timothy 4:1-5), depriving us of necessary minerals and vitamins, and offering substitutes that do more to ruin our health than animal fats ever could.
- Meat in moderation is a healthful and strength-building food.
- Health food stores sell beef, lamb, and fish that are free of synthetic hormones and antibiotics.
- Beef and other meats contain no more cholesterol than the same weight of fish fillets.[59]

IF YOUR CHOLESTEROL count is 220 or higher—the generally accepted level indicating increased susceptibility to heart attack—nutrition-oriented medical doctors recommend eating the following foods and taking vitamin supplements to lower blood cholesterol. (Rigorous exercise is also recommended.)

- Apples (one to three a day)
- Barley (several times a week in cereal or baked goods)
- Pinto or navy beans (a cup cooked each day)
- Carrots (three medium raw daily)
- Chili pepper (reduces blood serum cholesterol level by suppressing the liver's ability to produce cholesterol)
- Eggplant (blocks blood levels of cholesterol from rising when fatty foods have been eaten)
- Garlic (two to five cloves daily, or an odorless supplement)

- Grapefruit pectin (supplements)
- Lecithin (from soybeans and eggs, an ounce daily)
- Skim milk
- Oat bran (cereal or muffin)
- Olive oil (two teaspoons daily)
- Onions
- Green plantains
- Seafood (several times a week)
- Seaweed or kelp tablets
- Spinach
- Yams, sweet potatoes (four or five times a week)
- Yogurt (daily)
- Vitamin C (1,000-6,000 mg daily)[60]

DON'T USE POLYUNSATURATED oils! Researchers show they can cause premature aging, liver damage, lung deterioration, degeneration of the reproductive organs, and breast cancer.

- When polyunsaturated oils are heated, they become more saturated, said the former chairman of the Executive Committee of the National Safflower Council.
- Commercial varnish is produced by heating polyunsaturated oil.
- In scientific studies, varnish was an abnormal and dangerous by-product of the feces of animals who were fed heated polyunsaturated oils.
- Margarine is also unhealthful and void of nutritional value.[61]
- Polyunsaturated fatty-acids (PUFA) that are present in corn, safflower, sunflower, and peanut oil can destroy lung tissue and contribute to asthma.[62]

USE BUTTER OR olive oil—both of which are rich in nutrients—for cooking and baking (Isaiah 7:15). Always use any fatty food in moderation.[63]

HONEY—The most nutritious natural sweetener, you can get honey raw, unprocessed, and unfiltered. Use it instead of sugar.

- The Bible mentions honey as a wonderful food that must be eaten with wisdom and in moderation (Proverbs 25:16).
- Refined sugar in frequent high doses can cause diabetes, hypoglycemia, tooth decay, mental problems, learning disabilities, and a deficiency in vitamin B6.
- Sugar substitutes are just as dangerous as sugar. It's only a matter of time before you are totally saturated with chemical sweeteners and have to pay the price in your health.
- Honey is filled with minerals, helps with digestion, and prevents sore throats, colds, raw nerves, and insomnia.

YOU AND MEAT

PROTEIN IS ESSENTIAL for muscle growth and repair, proper healing, and sustained strength.

- Eat red meats no more than twice a week, poultry two or three times a week, and fish two times a week.
- No more than 25 percent of your total daily diet should be meat, fish, or dairy.
- Red meat digests slowly, so don't eat too much of it too often.

THE MEATS THAT Moses said were safe to eat have been proven to be the most healthy by scientists today.

- Beef and lamb come from animals that have cloven hooves and are, therefore, considered the healthiest of the meats (Leviticus 11:1-8).
- Meat from deer, elk, antelope, and moose (animals that have cloven hooves) is healthful and Biblically sound.
- Pigs are frequent carriers of highly dangerous parasites, such as trichinella spiralis (trichinosis), taenia solium (pork tapeworm), and disease-causing germs such as salmonella.

BEEF—It is all right to eat lean beef occasionally. Make it your feast food and limit your portions to 4 ounces.

EYE OF ROUND
- 243 calories per 3.5 ounces
- 14.2 grams fat

■ vitamin B12, niacin, folic acid
■ zinc, magnesium, potassium, iron

GROUND BEEF

■ 280 calories per 3.5 ounces broiled
■ 18.5 grams fat
■ folic acid, vitamin B12, niacin
■ magnesium, zinc, potassium, iron[64]

LAMB—Like other red meats, lamb is rich in B vitamins.

• The leg cut is the leanest and most tender, and tastes delicious when roasted. It is also perfect for stews.
• Jesus ate lamb at Passover and at the Last Supper (Luke 22:13-15).

■ 165 calories per 3 ounces leg roasted
■ 7 grams fat
■ niacin, riboflavin, thiamin
■ magnesium, zinc, potassium, iron[65]

CHICKEN—Experts say chicken and other poultry are ideal protein sources (Leviticus 11:20,21).

• Chicken is naturally rich in iron, niacin and zinc, and relatively low in saturated fat and sodium.
• Most chicken fat and calories are in the skin. New studies show you don't have to remove the skin before cooking— fat and cholesterol in the skin will impart a richer flavor but won't seep into the meat during the cooking process. Just remove the skin before eating to eliminate the bulk of saturated fats.
• Roasting is the healthiest and least caloric form of cooking.

■ 200 calories per 3.5 ounces
■ 4.5 grams fat
■ vitamin A, some B vitamins
■ magnesium, zinc, potassium, phosphorus, iron[66]

TURKEY—This poultry has one-fifth the amount of fat of beef in equal proportions.

■ 177 calories per 4 ounces

- 4 grams fat
- some B vitamins
- calcium, magnesium, zinc, potassium, iron[67]

DAIRY PRODUCTS

Have milk, unprocessed cheese, yogurt, cottage cheese, or butter at least 3 or 4 times a week.[68]

MILK—If available, try to get raw certified milk—its nutrients, minerals, and enzymes haven't been boiled out in the pasteurization process.[69]

- Milk and milk products should be taken in moderation.
- Some authorities recommend drinking whole milk, while others prefer skim. Since this debate has yet to be resolved, talk to the Lord about this and drink what you consider the best for you.
- Even skim milk, skim milk products, and non-fat yogurt are prime sources of calcium and protein.
- If you get cramps, gas, or diarrhea after drinking milk, you are intolerant of lactose, the sugar in milk.
- If you are intolerent, either cut out milk and milk products or get lactase (the enzyme that breaks down lactose) supplements at a health food store. (Yogurt doesn't bother the majority of people who are lactose intolerant.)[70]
- 86 calories per 8 ounces skim
- 0.4 grams fat
- vitamins A, D, some B vitamins
- calcium, potassium, magnesium, phosphorus[71]

YOGURT—Called *laban* in Bible times, yogurt has some extraordinary healing properties!

- Yogurt contains natural antibiotics and is excellent for intestinal infections and diarrhea, preventing or treating them.
- Yogurt can restore the normal balance of microbes in the bowels, which is necessary for proper digestion.

- It can lower blood cholesterol and boost the immune system.
- Don't buy sweetened yogurt, the kind with fruit added. Flavor it yourself with maple syrup, a teaspoon of instant coffee, or straight fruit conserves with no sugar added.
- Frozen yogurt, a highly processed food, doesn't count as yogurt.[72]
  - 127 calories per 8 oz. yogurt
  - 0.4 grams fat
  - vitamin A, some B vitamins
  - calcium, potassium, magnesium, zinc, phosphorus[73]

YOU AND FISH

FISH WAS ONE of the mainstays of the Bible diet, but some shellfish were toxic even back then (Leviticus 11:9-12).

- Fish contains rich oils which improve the cardiovascular system and prevent heart attacks.
- Shellfish often contains poisonous concentrations of mercury and other toxic metals and contaminants.
- Shrimp, lobster, oysters, and other shellfish are fine as occasional treats, but they should not be considered a "healthful" food.

STUDIES HAVE SHOWN that only one or two ounces of fish per day, or roughly two seafood meals a week, are enough to slash your risk of heart disease in half.

- Fish lowers your blood pressure and stimulates production of brain chemicals, making you more alert.
- Ocean fish contains a polyunsaturated oil called Omega 3 that protects against heart attacks and fatty acids.
- Omega 3 can thin the blood, insulate arteries from plaque build-up, dissolve dangerous clots, reduce dangerous triglycerides, decrease "bad" LDL cholesterol, diminish the risk of heart attacks and strokes, ease the symptoms of rheumatoid arthritis, lower the risk of lupus, protect against migraines, combat inflammation, tune up the immune

system, improve kidney function, fend off kidney disease, and relieve asthma.[74]

JESUS ATE FISH; He multiplied the two fish and five barley loaves for the multitude (Matthew 15:32-39), and He cooked and fed fish to several disciples, including Peter, after His resurrection (John 21:12,13).

- Jesus would only give you things that are good and healthful.

THE HIGHEST CONCENTRATIONS of Omega 3 oils are in extra-fatty fish such as mackerel, bluefish, tuna, sablefish, herring, anchovy, sardines, lake trout, pompano, sturgeon, and salmon.

- The best fish for health tend to be cold, saltwater fish, which live deep in the ocean.
- Commercially-cultivated fish raised in tanks or ponds, such as catfish, tend to be low in Omega 3. Much of the popular whitefish in the United States is relatively low in oil content.
  SALMON
  - 153 calories per 3 ounces waterpacked
  - 8.9 grams fat
  - vitamins A, some B vitamins
  - calcium, potassium
  TUNA
  - 158 calories per 3 ounces waterpacked
  - 6.9 grams fat
  - magnesium, potassium, phosphorus, iron[75]

FAST FOOD FISH filet sandwiches are a very poor source of seafood benefits! The National Institutes of Health's analysis shows most fast-food restaurants fry fish that are already low in Omega 3 oils in polyunsaturated oil (see subsection on polyunsaturated oil in this section) or animal fat.[76]

DIETARY SUPPLEMENTS

THE BIBLE DOESN'T mention vitamin or mineral supplements, but it does say that God wants His children to have abundant health

(Jeremiah 30:17; III John 2).

- Whether or not you take supplements is something you must discuss with your doctor to determine exactly which nutrients you need and in what amounts.
- When taken from natural sources, supplements put back into your body what is missing from your diet and necessary for your health.[77]
- Dietary supplements bring your body to the proper balance of digestive fluids, enzymes, vitamins, and minerals it needs to function properly.
- The body will use what it needs and excrete the rest. Some nutrients, such as copper and iodine, must be taken only in trace amounts available in food.[78]

IF YOU EAT nutritious foods in agreement with God's principles, you may not need food supplements.

- In today's world, eating fresh, natural food that hasn't been depleted of its nutrients is almost impossible.
- Improperly cooked and processed food may not deliver all the nutrients you need.
- A balanced combination of vitamins and minerals can reverse or prevent almost all common ailments and several severe diseases, such as cancer, heart disease, and diabetes.[79]

IF YOU TAKE supplements, be sure they are natural and pure.

- Don't use supplements that contain added chemicals.
- Read the labels![80]

FOLLOWING IS A partial list of vitamins and minerals that are essential to your health. If you are not receiving these nutrients through your diet, then you need supplements.

- If you eat junk food and try to make up for eating all those nutrient-depleted foods by taking supplements, you will not improve your health.
- Mineral and vitamin pills are meant to bolster an already nutritious diet.

BETA CAROTENE (Beta Carotene is converted into Vitamin A by the liver, except when you have liver trouble or a low thyroid function.)—dandelion greens, carrots, yams, kale, parsley, turnip greens, spinach, collard greens, chard, watercress, red peppers, squash, cantaloupe, endive, persimmons, apricots, broccoli, pimentos, mangoes, papayas, nectarines, pumpkins, peaches, cherries, lettuce, tomatoes, asparagus, soybeans, kumquats, watermelon[81]

CALCIUM—sesame seeds, kelp, cheese, brewer's yeast, torula yeast, parsley, Brazil nuts, watercress, salmon, chickpeas, eggs, beans, pistachios, lentils, kale, sunflower seeds, dairy products, buckwheat, maple syrup, chard, walnuts, spinach, endive, pecans, wheat germ, peas, peanuts, oats[82]

FOLIC ACID—torula yeast, brewer's yeast, alfalfa, soybeans, endive, chickpeas, oats, lentils, beans, wheat germ, liver, split peas, whole wheat, barley, brown rice, asparagus, green peas, sunflower seeds, collard greens, spinach, hazelnuts, kale, peanuts, soy lecithin, walnuts, corn, Brussels sprouts, broccoli, Brazil nuts, almonds[83]

IRON (Athletes and women especially need this nutrient, and everyone needs at least 500 mg. Iron is best absorbed when taken with vitamin C-rich foods like orange juice, oranges, or the supplement itself.)—blackstrap molasses, brown rice, chickpeas, dried apricots, meat, nuts, raisins, walnuts, wheat bran, white beans[84]

MAGNESIUM (It is needed to control high blood pressure.[85] Taken with zinc, magnesium can eliminate difficult body odor.[86] It can also be used as treatment for bedwetting.)[87]—kelp, blackstrap molasses, sunflower seeds, wheat germ, almonds, soybeans, Brazil nuts, bone meal, pistachio nuts, soy lecithin, hazelnuts, pecans, oats, walnuts, brown rice, chard, spinach, barley, coconut, salmon, corn, avocados, bananas, cheese, tuna, potatoes, cashews, turkey[88]

POTASSIUM (This nutrient is essential for heart health.)—beans, parsley, peas, pistachios, wheat germ, sunflower seeds, chickpeas, almonds, seasame seeds, Brazil nuts, peanuts, pecans[89]

PROTEIN—cheese, eggs, fish, meat, milk, soy flour, tofu, yeast and yogurt, legumes, grain, nuts and seeds, dark leafy greens[90]

RIBOFLAVIN—dairy products, eggs, whole and enriched grains, brewer's yeast, dark leafy greens, legumes[91]

SELENIUM (Take this supplement ONLY under a doctor's care. It is a trace mineral that works with vitamin E to combat breast cysts, and may be helpful in preventing breast cancer.)[92]—corn, cabbage, whole wheat, beans, peas, vegetable oils, onions, chicken, beets, barley, tomatoes, soybeans, saltwater fish, freshwater fish, liver, seaweed, brown rice, alfalfa, peanuts[93]

VITAMIN B6—brewer's yeast, brown rice, whole wheat, soybeans, rye, lentils, sunflower seeds, hazelnuts, alfalfa, salmon, wheat germ, tuna, bran, walnuts, peas, liver, avocados, beans, cashews, peanuts, oats, beef, chicken, turkey, halibut, lamb, banana, blackstrap molasses, corn, eggs[94]

VITAMIN B12 (Supplements of this vitamin are critically necessary if you are a strict vegetarian. A deficiency can lead to pernicious anemia; it is hard to digest for vegetarians, so get a supplement that has "intrinsic factor," which makes it more readily assimilated.)[95]—lamb and beef [and especially the organ meats of cows and sheep—liver, kidneys, heart, sweetbreads], clams, oysters, sardines, trout, salmon, lobster, scallops, haddock, flounder, swordfish, halibut, perch, tuna, Brie, Camembert and Limburger cheeses, dairy products, eggs, nutritional yeast[96]

VITAMIN C (Take between 1,000 and 5,000 mg daily, but start out at lower doses as vitamin C supplements may make you nauseous at first. You need a supplement unless you are getting more than 1,000 mg a day through food—four ounces of acerola cherries, four ounces or rose hips [the ripe fruit of a rose], or 80 ounces of spinach. This vitamin is an important antioxidant, which keeps muscles and bones strong, strengthens the adrenal and immune systems, and protects against infection and degeneration.)[97]—rose hips, acerola cherries, guavas, black currants, parsley, green peppers, watercress, chives, strawberries, persimmons, spinach, oranges, cabbage, grapefruit, papaya, elderberries, kumquats, dandelion greens, lemons, cantaloupe, green onions, limes, mangoes, loganberries, tangerines, tomatoes, squash, raspberries, romaine lettuce, pineapple[98]

VITAMIN D—cod liver oil, sardines, salmon, tuna, eggs, sunflower seeds, liver, butter, cheese, cream, corn oil, milk, cottage cheese[99]

VITAMIN E (Supplements of 600 IU of vitamin E are needed daily to combat fibrocystic disease, or cysts in the breasts. It must be taken with vitamin A to assure proper assimilation.)[100]—wheat germ, safflower nuts, sunflower seeds, whole wheat, sesame oil, walnuts, hazelnuts, almonds, olive oil, cabbage, Brazil nuts, peanuts, cod liver oil, cashews, soy lecithin, spinach, asparagus, broccoli, butter, parsley, oats, barley, corn, avocados[101]

ZINC—herring (especially rich, with 110 mg per four ounces), liver, sesame seeds, soybeans, lamb, chicken, oats, rye, wheat, corn, eggs, cheese, legumes, nuts, wheat germ, whole grains, some kinds of brewer's yeast[102]

Section Two
HEALTHY APPETITES FOR A LONG LIFE

Food was a very spiritual thing in the Old and New Testaments. Eating was not just something the Israelites casually did; it had to do with their covenant relationship with God. Meals indicated the making or renewing of covenants. The Israelites prayed over their food before and after each meal because food to them was a spiritual encounter with God.

We've misconstrued eating in today's society, and consequently the thing that God intended to bless and sustain us has become a curse for many. Eating should reflect our covenant relationship with our heavenly Father. The New Testament says we are to receive our food with thanksgiving, sanctified (or set apart) by prayer. With a fast food restaurant on almost every corner, I think it would be safe to say that few of us view food or our mealtimes as anything holy unto the Lord.

There is a definite renewing of covenant in food, and if we would view our fellowship and meals in that respect, we would be able to get our appetites in line with the Word of God.

BIBLE FOODS THAT ARE HEALTHY

WE NEED TO know the "truth" about God's Word in the area of eating so that we are not "... *carried about with every wind of doctrine ...* " (Ephesians 4:14).

- God had a great purpose in giving Moses the dietary laws that we read about in the Old Testament. He wanted the Israelites to maintain a right relationship with Him and to trust Him for their food.
- He also wanted a healthy people free from contamination. He told them to do some things that are kind of unusual

to us . . . things that nutritionist are now telling us are "right on."

I HAVE LEARNED a way of eating that is simple, balanced, and easy to understand.

- It is a "way of life for eating"; not a diet.
- It is the way to eat whether you need to gain or lose weight, remain the same, or get well.
- That way is eating food the way God made it—PURE![1]

THE KEY TO good health is to keep your blood clean through proper foods; exercise; plenty of water; fasting and prayer; fresh air and sunshine; and peaceful, stress-free living.

- Eating food the way God made it cleanses the blood from impurities by supplying it with all the nutrients necessary to rebuild cells.
- The Lord's way of eating will keep your blood clean and healthy, which will automatically protect you from infection.
  - ■ A dirty blood stream is the main cause of illness and premature aging.
- When the bloodstream is pure it will dissolve all poisons and carry them away.

KEEPING THE BLOODSTREAM clean, and the body healthy, requires personal discipline.

- You must supervise what goes into your stomach.
- The human body can take years of punishment before it rebels against being loaded down with foodless foods and the poisons they produce.
- When the body cannot undo the damage done to it fast enough, the bloodstream becomes clogged and dirty.
- The whole system begins to break down and becomes a breeding ground for disease, which results in premature aging.[2]

CERTAIN FOODS DESTROY our health and fill our body with poisons.

- Chemical preservatives, artificial flavors and colors, and synthetic vitamins have been added to our foods to make them more attractive, quick to prepare, and stable for years on the grocery shelf.

- We are sick and overweight because we eat more refined food than natural, pure food.[3]

ONLY PURE FOOD is life-giving.

- Foods that aren't natural will always interfere with your body's function in some way.
- Natural foods promote health, strength, endurance and long life; whereas processed foods promote disease and death.

THE SAME IS true for the food God made.

- The more processes it goes through before it gets to your body, the less it will have to offer.
- When you eat refined, processed, devitalized foods, your body isn't nourished and you don't feel satisfied; so you overeat to make up for it. (see I Corinthians 10:23; II Corinthians 7:1).

GOD HAS A divine way for you to eat so that you might have divine health.

- Your body is the temple of the Lord and you should respect and honor it (I Corinthians 3:16,17).

GOD TOLD ADAM and Eve to eat seed that grew on the trees, fruit, and vegetables (see Genesis 1:29).[4]

- God did not permit man to eat meat until after the flood (Genesis 9:3).

EIGHT BIBLE HEALTH FOODS

AN APPLE A day keeps the doctor away.

- Apples are good for you because they contain a concentrated amount of pectin, a highly soluble fiber.
- Soluble fibers absorb water in the large intestine, adding bulk to waste matter and softening it.
- Apples prevent irritation of the colon, which can lead to ailments including hemorrhoids and cancer.

- The high fiber content makes them excellent for the control of blood sugar and the prevention and treatment of diabetes.
- Apples help curb the appetite.
- If you eat two apples a day you can lower your total cholesterol level, and in some cases elevate the good cholesterol level.

BARLEY STICKS TO your ribs and prevents you from gaining weight.

- It is very nutritious and raises the level of good cholesterol.
- Barley is one of the healthiest grains.
- Only the poorest Israelites ate barley because it was inexpensive.
  - The Israelites almost always had longer life spans, and more energy and strength than their masters (see GUIDELINES FOR HEALTHY EATING.)

GARLIC, LEEKS, AND RADISHES historically have been used to ward off infection.

- People who eat lots of garlic rarely have colds.

LENTILS ARE AN extremely mineral-rich bean.

- Because they are small and easy to travel with, they were used a lot in Old Testament times.
- Esau loved lentils so much that he sold his birthright for a bowl of them.

WHEAT RAISES ALL levels of good cholesterol.

- All of your vitamin B complexes can be found in wheat and other grains.

TWO HELPINGS OF fish a week will slash the risk of heart disease in half.

- Fish cleanses the blood stream, thins the blood, insulates the arteries from plaque build up, dissolves clots, reduces triglycerides (dangerous fat), lowers LDL cholesterol, diminishes the risk of heart attacks and strokes, eases the symptoms of rheumatoid arthritis, lowers the risk of lupus, protects against migraines, combats inflammation, tunes up the immune system, improves kidney functions, fends off kidney diseases, and relieves asthma.

- What makes fish so valuable is its oil content, which is full of Omega 3 fatty acids (oils found in fish that lower the level of LDL cholesterol in your bloodstream).

HONEY IS A predigested food and is easier on your body to digest.

- Because honey is predigested, it is very nutritious to your body.
- Honey is a natural energy source.
- Jonathan tasted honey and his eyes were enlightened (I Samuel 14:25-27).

LAMB IS EXTREMELY rich in B vitamins.

- Lamb was the Passover meat.

JESUS WAS **NOT** a vegetarian.

- Jesus ate lamb during the Passover and honeycomb and fish after His resurrection.
- Although Jesus ate meat, people did not consume meat in large quantities during Biblical times.
- Americans today eat meat at almost every meal.
- Nutritionists warn that consuming large quantities of meat will shorten your life span.

YOU DO NOT have to be a vegetarian to be healthy and to maintain a covenant relationship with God.

- *"Forbidding to marry, and commanding to abstain from meats, which God hath created to be received with thanksgiving of them which believe and know the truth. For every creature of God is good, and nothing to be refused, if it be received with thanksgiving: for it is sanctified by the word of God and prayer"* (I Timothy 4:3-5).
- Every **creature** is good for food.
  - Remember, though, you are not to be riotous eaters of flesh (Proverbs 23:20).

ASK GOD TO bless and sanctify your food and He will take away sickness from you (Deuteronomy 7:13-15).

- You can't always be extremely selective about what you eat, but you can pray the right thing over your food before you eat it.

WHAT YOU PRAY over is set apart by the Lord for your well-being.

- If nutrition is lacking in what you have to eat, God can make it up to you if you will sanctify it with prayer (see YOUR FOOD ATTITUDES FOR HEALTHY LIVING).
- That *doesn't* mean you can neglect good meal planning. You may be in a position sometimes where you can't eat correctly.

LOOSING THE BANDS OF WICKEDNESS

FASTING LOOSES THE bands of wickedness.

- Like food, fasting is a spiritual discipline unto the Lord.
- To fast means "to abstain from all or certain foods."
- Fasting is a discipline God designed to bring you into a greater knowledge of Him, to release you into more fullness and power of the Holy Spirit's work in your life, and to bring you to a point of greater health.[5]

FASTING CAN ALTER your life in such a way that you are free to move in new freedom, new closeness to God, and new unity with your fellow man.

- Shutting down the body and giving it a break from all the heavy food you consume is like giving the body a "new beginning."
- Fasting is a personal matter between you and God—an offering to Him.
- Fasting should be approached prayerfully and by the leading of the Holy Spirit (Matthew 6:17,18).

A GOD KIND of fast will "... *loose the bands of wickedness, undo the heavy burdens, ... let the oppressed go free, and ... break every yoke*" (Isaiah 58:6).

- Fasting is deliberately denying yourself food for a set period of time in order to give yourself more completely to prayer and closer communication with God.[6]

THE SPIRITUAL SIDE of fasting is far more significant than the physical.

- Fasting is a cleansing process from beginning to end. It cleanses your spirit, soul, mind, and body all at the same time.

- Physically our bodies are constantly eliminating poisons through the lungs, skin, bowels, and kidneys; and fasting provides the most favorable conditions under which to accomplish these things.

WHEN YOU FAST, the body is free to do what it does best, which is a natural self-healing and cleansing process.

- Because you abstain from food while fasting, the energy normally used to digest, assimilate, and metabolize your food is now spent purifying the body.
- Fasting cleanses the bloodstream.
- Premature aging is arrested.
- Fasting causes you to look more attractive; and to feel better physically, mentally, and spiritually.
- Your spirit, soul, and body become cleaner and purer with each day of your fast.
  - Fasting is a very quick way to bring about a release of toxins from the body.

FASTING IS A time of rest, rejuvenation, and cleansing.

- Because fasting cleanses your body of toxins, when you feel a minor illness coming on, a fast can sometimes prevent its development by allowing the body to concentrate on the self-healing and cleansing processes.

THE CLEANER YOU become internally the more you will desire food the way God made it and the less you will have a taste for low-quality or junk food.[7]

- The cleaner you become in your spirit, the less attracted

you will be to anything of a polluted, perverted, or unclean nature.

FASTING, PHYSICAL EXERCISE, and eating food the way God made it are the keys to healthy weight loss.

- A low-calorie diet is torture. Fasting is not.
- Extreme calorie-restricted diets are unnatural. Fasting is ordained by God.
- Fasting helps to balance out your weight.[8]

IN A SOCIETY where eating is the "in thing" to do, some individuals struggle to maintain their weight.

- They have too small an appetite and eat too little.
- Many studies indicate that appetite loss can be caused by
  - Eating too little to supply the nutrients which tend to generate hunger
  - Inability to experience the full range of tastes
  - Prescription drugs
  - Celiac disease (a condition which prevents the absorption of fat and calcium) which is often treated with apples and banana pulp

HELP FOR A POOR APPETITE

IN THE EVENT of too little food intake, appetite can be increased by increasing the consumption of the best supplements and food sources of vitamins B1 and B12.

- Inability to taste and smell properly limits the appetite and desire to eat.
- This food deficiency usually results from insufficient food intake to supply all the necessary nutrients.[9]

THE ABUSES OF EATING

THE ABUSE OF eating normally occurs because Jesus is not Lord

at the table.
- Commit your appetite to Him.

ELI WAS VERY, very fat.
- He ate the fat of the sacrifices.
- He was overindulgent in the area of his appetite and with his children.
- His overindulgence with his children caused his family's downfall.
- Though the Lord warned him to get his house in order, Eli refused and his children died prematurely and did not inherit the promises of God (I Samuel 2,3).

LUSTING AFTER FOOD is another abuse of eating.
- It is natural to have a desire for food.
  - ■ Your body requires food to sustain you.

KEEP YOUR MIND and body busy (Proverbs 27:7).
- If you examine the times in which you crave certain foods, you'll discover it's when you are idle.
  - ■ Idleness can best be described as a period of time when you don't have much to do (Proverbs 19:15).
- A mind that is full, complete, and constantly thinking about worthwhile things won't make periodic stops at the refrigerator.
- People with full souls and occupied minds are not thinking about sweets all the time—they are too busy filling their minds with thoughts of achievement.

THE BIBLE TELLS you how to handle your cravings.
- Confess the Word about your health AND modify your behavior.
- Change your eating habits (I Corinthians 10:31).

THE HUNGRY SOUL, or the person whose mind is idle and undisciplined, thinks that everything tastes good.
- Another key to eating properly is found in Proverbs 13:25: *"The righteous eateth to the satisfying of his soul: but the belly of the wicked shall want."*

- ■ The important word here is *satisfying*. You can eat to the satisfying of your soul or you can go beyond that amount and stuff yourself.
- Most people go beyond being satisfied because the food tastes **so** good.
- The righteous don't go beyond being satisfied; they stay within that limit.

GOD HAS GIVEN you only *one* body for this life.

- If you abuse it, you will shorten your life span.
- Glorify God with your mind, emotions, and body.

OVEREATING IS ANOTHER form of eating abuse and is often the result of psychological problems and hurts.

- If you are guilty of this, try to discern the reason why.
- Many people overeat in times of major change, extreme stress, disappointment, busyness, or during certain illnesses.
- The worst part about overeating is that you normally overeat food that has no nourishment.
  - ■ You end up eating even more to make up for the hidden hunger or empty, incomplete feeling.
- Much eating is merely catering to out-of-control taste buds rather than to real hunger.

OVEREATING OVERTAXES THE digestive organs because the body can't process the food fast enough.

- It makes the stomach, liver, kidneys, and bowels work harder than they are supposed to work.
- If the food cannot be processed before it putrefies, poisons from the purification are absorbed into the blood and the whole system is affected by dirty blood and poisons.
- Overeating uses up your energy supply.
- If all you feel like doing after a meal is taking a nap, it could be that you are eating too much.
- You can overeat good food as well as junk food.
- Always remember, even food that is good for you, consumed in excess, can be harmful.[10]

DO YOUR EATING habits glorify God?

- You can be **skinny** and still not glorify God in your eating habits.
- Proverbs 23:2 says to *". . . put a knife to thy throat, if thou be a man given to appetite."*

ONE OF THE best ways to handle a bad eating habit is to pray in the Spirit (Romans 8:26).

- The Spirit will help you when you are weak.
- Pray for ten minutes before you begin to eat.
- Pray in the Spirit when you pass the refrigerator.
- Praying in the Spirit will help you in your area of weakness and turn it into one of your areas of strength.

CONTROL YOUR SUGAR CONSUMPTION

SUGAR CONSUMPTION SEEMS to be a big problem in our nation.

- Craving for sweets is probably a direct result of having been rewarded with something sweet as a child.
- Refined sugar is bad for you.
- Refined sugar in frequent high doses can cause diabetes, hypoglycemia, tooth decay, mental problems, learning disabilities, and B vitamin complex shortage.
    - Sugar substitutes are just as dangerous as sugar.[11]
    - Honey, if overdone, can be harmful as well.

EAT WHAT YOU know you are comfortable with and don't overdo it (Proverbs 25:16).

- A lot of people contract diseases in their older years because they ate too much sugar when they were younger.
- Sugar not only destroys the physical body, but it also adversely affects the mind.

HONEY IS THE most nutritious natural sweetener you can get

if you buy it "raw," "unprocessed," and "unfiltered."
- Throughout the Bible honey is mentioned as a wonderful food to be used with wisdom and in balance.
- Honey is filled with minerals and is an aid to digestion.
- It also helps to prevent sore throats, colds, raw nerves, and insomnia.[12]

NUTRITION, RELATIONSHIPS, AND DISEASE

MANY ARTICLES ON nutrition say good nutrition can save marriages, reduce crime, empty the mental hospitals, and generally make us better persons.
- The answer to these problems is not diet alone, but poor nutrition probably does exacerbate the problem.

SOME EXPERTS IN the field say that people carry between five and twenty pounds of toxins and wastes inside of them.
- If all those poisons aren't released, your body will break down under the stress and become sick, and your personal relationships can be affected.

TOXIC WASTES BUILD up in your body when you eat too many impure, processed, foodless foods and don't give your body a chance to rest and get rid of them.
- The body will try to cleanse itself naturally.

DISEASE DOESN'T COME overnight; it builds for a long time.
- To take the mystery out of being sick, think of disease as another way of saying "out of balance."
- Poisons will settle quickly wherever you have a weak area in your body.
- A weak area will flare up again and again: the same sinus condition, stomach problem, aching shoulder, or just plain crummy feeling. These are some of the indications that you have a toxic buildup.[13]

GOD CAN REFRESH and revitalize our bodies. The Bible says Christians are going to live longer than sinners—we don't smoke, drink, take drugs. We don't do a lot of things sinners do.

- Our bodies can be renewed even when we have abused them.
- If God can renew our minds, He can renew our bodies.

ANOREXIA

ANOREXIA DESTROYS THE human body.

- Anorexics are so intent on losing weight, they literally starve themselves to death.
  - One-third of all anorexic victims (mainly young girls) die.
- Anorexics are now classified as psychotics, not neurotics.
- This condition is commonly attributed to a zinc deficiency which can reduce appetite, mainly by diminishing the ability to taste and smell foods to the fullest extent.
- Researchers are uncertain if a zinc deficiency causes anorexia or whether it is just related to the disorder's symptoms.
- The appropriate nutrient for anorexia nervosa is 50 milligrams of zinc sulfate, three times a day with meals.
- Zinc makes a positive contribution to coping with anorexia nervosa.[14]

BULIMIA

BULIMIA IS CHARACTERIZED by binge-eating, then vomiting or using cathartics or diuretics.

- "Bulimia" actually means *ox* or *bull hunger.*
- An estimated 30 percent of all high school and college girls use this method to stabilize their weight.
- Statistics indicate that 19 percent of all women and five percent of all men are bulimic.
- Underlying this desperate measure is a personality plagued

by emotional stress: frustration, emptiness, feelings of low self-esteem, self-consciousness, loneliness, depression and perfectionism.

THE SIGNS OF bulimia include

- Disappearance to the bathroom soon after eating
- A faint odor of gastric juices from throwing up, despite a mouthwash
- A constant, strong cover-up odor
- A puffy face
- Irregular menstrual cycles or the absence of them
- A sore throat from the food's two-way traffic
- Mottled or stained teeth (erosion from powerful gastric juices)
- Hair loss (caused by insufficient key nutrients and emotional stress)

THE RANKIN METHOD has been used to treat bulimics.

- It combines psychology with some nutrition.
- Its primary focus is changing the bulimic's behavior, not curing symptoms.

EATING HABITS ARE learned habits.

- You can teach yourself to eat any way you want.
- You learned to love the foods you love now; you can learn to love God's food just as much.[15]

HELPFUL HINTS

1) When choosing food always ask yourself: "Is this man-made or God-made?" and "How pure can I get it?"
2) The fewer items in a meal, the less you are tempted to overeat and the easier it is to digest.
3) The more natural the food, the more healthful it is, and the harder it is for you to overeat.
4) The less active your life or work, the less you need to eat.
5) Space your eating to five or six hours between each meal (unless otherwise advised by your doctor).

6) Each week, eliminate from your diet one or two foods on the foods-to-avoid list and add from the foods-to-include list.

7) Don't eat an excess of overcooked or processed foods.

8) Eat foods ripe and in season.

9) Drink water, herb teas, and freshly squeezed juices.

10) Don't eat fried food.

11) Eat simply and plainly.

12) Never overeat.

13) Chew well.

14) Read labels.

15) At least fifty percent of every meal should consist of raw or properly cooked fruits and vegetables.

FRUITS AND VEGETABLES are eliminating and cleansing foods, and are alkaline forming.

- Starches and proteins are body builders, and are acid forming.
- You always want a more alkaline body. A too acidic condition breeds disease.
- Poisons move out of the body when raw or properly cooked fruits and vegetables are eaten.

SET ASIDE THREE special times of the year for a week of cleansing.

- Begin with a three-day fast and then eat only a wide variety of fresh fruits and vegetables for a few days after that.
- The best times of the year for this are
    - January, after Christmas and New Year's celebrations are over
    - Late spring (May is good) to prepare you for the seasonal change to summer (you'll have more resistance to colds)
    - September, when you're about to change your style of living again from summer to fall

A STRICT DIET of fresh fruits and vegetables may not seem fun but you'll find it is a lot more fun than being sick (Daniel 1:12-15).

- If you have a problem eating fruit, stick with vegetables until your body balances itself.

- When you go on a cleansing diet you may find that you have a headache, chills, or diarrhea, or what seems like hay fever or a slight cold. Don't be alarmed; it is just poison coming out of your system.
- Drink plenty of water and pure herb teas to help flush out the body.
- You may find that your whole mental attitude and outlook will change when you are free from poisons in your system.

MANY DIETARY ELEMENTS are necessary to produce good health.

- If you do not want to sit down with charts and a calculator at each meal to see if you are getting everything you need, then read GUIDELINES FOR HEALTHY LIVING.[16]

FRIED FOODS ARE hard to digest.

- Frying destroys a lot of the vitamins and minerals in food.
  - Some authorities say oil becomes carcinogenic when heated to a high temperature, so don't make fried foods your way of life.
  - If you're in a restaurant or someone's home when fried food is served—or if you have been good for a month and just want a hamburger and french fries—then go ahead and enjoy it.[17]

WHATEVER YOU DO only now and then in your eating habits, whether it is something good for you or something bad, won't make much difference in the long run.

- It's what you do every day that determines whether you will be healthy or sick.

DON'T MAKE YOUR diet meat-heavy.

- Only 25% of your diet should be meat.
  - Too much meat can be exhausting for your system to process and the result may be fatigue and weight gain.[18]

HERBAL TEA HAS a soothing and healing quality to it.

- Herbs have been used as medicine since Adam and Eve.

- When you are healthy you won't need something as strong and stimulating as coffee to get you going.
- Herbal tea is also good after meals because it aids in digestion.[19]

FOODS TO AVOID

1) White sugar
2) White-sugar products (jams, jelly, prepared gelatin desserts, cakes, candies, cookies, pies, pudding, fruits canned in sugar, etc.)
3) White flour
4) White-flour products (macaroni, noodles, spaghetti)
5) Wheat flour—usually a mixture of white and wheat—should say whole wheat or stone-ground whole wheat
6) Soft drinks made with sugar and chemicals
7) Refined cereals
8) Salt and highly salted foods (potato chips, salted nuts, pretzels, olives, etc.)
9) White rice
10) Hydrogenated oils and saturated fats
11) Peanut butter—made from saturated fats and hydrogenated oils
12) Margarine made from saturated fats and hydrogenated oils
13) Heavily processed meats (hot dogs, salami, bologna, bacon, corned beef, etc.)
14) Canned goods that contain white flour, sugar, or chemicals
15) Chocolate
16) Ice cream made with chemicals
17) Coffee, tea, and alcohol
18) "Instant" packaged foods
19) Fried foods
20) Canned fruits and vegetables

FOODS TO INCLUDE

1) Honey or at least unrefined sugar used sparingly
2) Foods sweetened with honey (other good sweeteners are blackstrap molasses, fruit, fruit juice, dates)
3) Whole-grain flour (barley, oats, wheat, millet, rye, buckwheat, etc.)
4) Whole-grain products (noodles, macaroni, etc., made with sesame, soya, whole wheat)
5) Whole-wheat flour or any other whole-grain flour mixture
6) Natural fruit juices (if you must have soft drinks, at least buy the natural ones like grapefruit soda, lemon-lime soda, sparkling apple juice, etc.)
7) Whole-grain cereal (raw oats, four-grain cereal, whole-grain granola, etc.)
8) Natural vegetable seasonings (instead of salt)
9) Natural brown rice (also unprocessed wild rice)
10) Oils that are naturally pressed and unrefined especially sesame, corn, safflower, soya, all-blend oils
11) Natural peanut butter made without chemicals, heavy processing, and salt
12) Butter made as purely as possible
13) Pure meats (look for all-meat hot dogs, bacon, etc., that are made without chemicals, sugar, preservatives, and heavy spices)
14) Canned goods that are pure (natural ingredients)
15) Carob
16) Ice cream made with pure foods such as pure milk, eggs, and honey
17) Herbal teas
18) Natural unprocessed products (i.e., real potatoes as opposed to instant)
19) Baked, poached, steamed, or stewed foods
20) Fresh fruits and vegetables[20]

YOUR FOOD ATTITUDES FOR HEALTHY LIVING

OVEREATING: THE ABUSE OF YOUR BODY

OVEREATING WILL AFFECT your body, the way you think, the way you act, and even your self-image.

- Overeating will make you overweight.
- People who are overweight have a much greater risk of dying prematurely than people of normal weight.
- God did not create you to be sick and die prematurely.

IF YOU ARE born again, you have eaten with the Lord Jesus Christ.

- You have eaten of His flesh spiritually and you have drunk of His blood spiritually.
- You have entered into a covenant relationship and cannot treat your body any way you want and indulge your appetite because you do not belong to yourself anymore.
- You were bought with a price.
- Your body must be directed by Him.
- Ask yourself, "Will people see God in me when I overeat and am overweight?"

WHEN YOU EAT more food than your body can use—even on a nutritionally sound diet—you will become overweight.

- Overeating is never good for you at any time and is especially harmful as a way of life.
- When you overeat, you are abusing and misusing your body.
- When you overeat, the body can't process the food fast

enough, and your digestive organs (stomach, liver, kidneys, and bowels) have to work harder than they should.[1]

- Not enough digestive enzymes can be sent to the stomach for massive (or even slightly large) amounts of food, so some of the food remains undigested.
- Undigested food rots, breeding unwelcome bacteria in your bowels, sending toxins in your blood, and creating foul breath, body odors, and intestinal gas.[2]

BEING GROSSLY OVERWEIGHT or oven moderately heavy can cause a variety of diseases, including heart and artery problems, high blood pressure, diabetes, cancer, and more.

- If you are overweight, repent of your sin of overeating and not exercising, ask God to forgive and help you, and change your lifestyle.
- You cannot treat your overeating and/or extra weight flippantly.

EVEN IF YOU have limited abdominal obesity, you should not be complacent.

- Any oversize paunch in your abdominal area could be hazardous.
  - To check whether you are at risk, measure your waist and hips with a tape measure. If your waist is larger than your hips, you better start reducing!
- An enlarged belly brings a tremendous risk of heart disease, stroke, and diabetes.
- Fatty tissue in the stomach floods the liver with fatty acids and interferes with the liver's ability to control blood levels of insulin, leading to diabetes.
- Abdominal fat can interfere with menstrual cycles by limiting the production of insulin.
- Dieting and regular aerobic exercise can help get rid of your oversized belly and reduce the risk of health problems.[3]

EXTRA WEIGHT ON any part of your body leads to disease.

- Stress, overweight, and lack of exercise set you up for back injury.

- People who are obese subject their limbs to unusual uses and stress, causing osteoarthritis (an ailment that disintegrates the cartilage in the joints).
- Obesity can cause diabetes.
  - The longer you are overweight, the less insulin your body will deliver to your muscles, which will take up less energy-giving glucose.
  - The more fat you carry, the more tissue area your pancreas has to service, making it impossible to produce enough insulin to meet your entire body's demands.[4]
  - When body fat competes with muscle for insulin, the fat wins, turning the carbohydrates you eat into still more fat.
  - A high-fiber diet, full of raw fruits and vegetables, nuts, seeds, and whole grains will help control the problem.
  - Losing weight will control and may even eliminate this type of diabetes.[5]
- People who are grossly overweight and even those who are marginally overweight can experience raised cholesterol and triglyceride (dangerous fat) levels, which will contribute to high blood pressure.
  - The heart must pump blood through two miles of extra arteries for each pound of fat.
  - Obesity and high blood pressure encourage congestive heart failure, arterial disease, and sudden death.
  - Losing weight will help reduce blood pressure because you will relieve the stress on the heart, which rests only between beats.
  - A predisposition to obesity-caused high blood pressure is often passed on to your children.[6]
- The American Cancer Society says overweight people have an increased risk of breast, colon, gallbladder, kidney, stomach, and uterine cancer.[7]
  - Overweight women are at greater risk of developing cancer

than overweight men.

■ Obesity doesn't cause breast cancer, but it encourages its spread.

■ Obesity contributes to prostate cancer in men.[8]

• Pregnancy is complicated by obesity, which causes toxemia, diabetes mellitus (a type of diabetes occurring during pregnancy that may continue for the rest of the mother's life), and varicose veins; and obesity increases the need for caesarean sections.[9]

• Overweight and diabetic men may become impotent.[10]

• Overweight men and women may become infertile.[11]

• Obesity causes gallbladder trouble.[12]

• People who are overweight will have difficulty breathing because fat restricts chest expansion.

■ Unless you lose weight, this condition becomes worse with time because the pressure of fat limits lung capacity, air flow, and exhalation of carbon dioxide.[13]

• Overeating and obesity can contribute to liver malfunction and damage.

■ Damage to the liver, the body's enzyme factory, limits its ability to create enough energy-producing enzymes.

■ When enzymes aren't produced, fuel cannot be burned up fast enough so that fat accumulates.

■ The liver will regenerate itself if you go on a pure, nutritious, sensible diet, and you get plenty of exercise.[14]

GET YOUR APPETITE IN LINE

OVEREATING CAN BE caused by the lack of something in your life.

• Food has become a substitute for what is missing in your life or is used to comfort you.

• Jesus can set you free.

• Don't run from your appetite problem—run to God with it.

- When you lay your appetite at the Cross, He will help you.

DON'T THINK YOU are helpless or hopeless because your appetite has hurt your body and has taken over your life.

- God sent His Son to save a world of sinners (John 3:16).
- He doesn't deny anyone salvation, blessings, or healing, no matter his or her past (Romans 8:38,39).
- By Christ's stripes you are healed (I Peter 2:24).

THERE ARE THREE kinds of Christians—spiritual, soulish, and carnal.

- When awakened from a sound slumber at 2 a.m. with a craving to eat the rest of last night's fried chicken, these three Christians will act differently.
    - The spiritual Christian, who is led by the Holy Spirit, will say, "That appetite is out of line; Lord, I want to submit my appetite to You. I want You to guide me and direct my mind, my thinking, and my body. My body belongs to You. My body doesn't belong to me."
    - The soulish Christian, who considers his intellect higher than the Word of God, says, "Wait a minute. It's not good to eat at 2 a.m. or to eat all that fried food. I better go back to bed."
    - The carnal Christian, who puts his flesh above God, says, "I'll need some mashed potatoes and gravy with that chicken."
- What kind of Christian are you?

SEEK GOD'S HELP to control your appetite.

- Repent of your destructive behavior.
- Commit your appetite into God's hands.
- Accept God's grace and forgiveness.
- Take His power to set you free and help you walk in that freedom.
- Pray this wonderful Scripture: *"Lord, feed me with food that is convenient for me"* (Proverbs 30:8).
- Praying in the Spirit will help you overcome your weakness

and turn it into an area of strength (Romans 8:26).
- Pray in the Spirit for 10 minutes before you eat.
- Pray in the Spirit before you pass the refrigerator or any time you are tempted.
- Through incessant eating you have made food an idol.
  - When you place food above God and your relationship with Him, food is an idol.
  - Put God first in ALL things (Exodus 20:2-5).

FOR AN EXTREMELY difficult appetite problem, Proverbs 23:2 says to put a knife to your throat, **figuratively speaking,** of course.
- God is serious about your appetite because when you are out-of-control, you will die prematurely.
- Jesus told you to cut off your right hand if it offends you to show you that your body is not more important than your obedience to God (Matthew 5:30).
- Your body is the temple of God and is holy (I Corinthians 3:16,17).
- God wants you to finish what He has called you to do (Hebrews 12:1).

EAT WITH TEMPERANCE (see Proverbs 25:16).
- Eat only what your body can handle, only what is sufficient (Proverbs 30:8).
- Get your eyes off physical food and be fed with what is really necessary for your body, soul, and spirit—God's Word.

IDENTIFY THE FOODS you crave the most.
- Find out why you eat too fast, too much, between meals, when you're unhappy, when you're alone, etc.
- Good food will satisfy you and meet all your body's needs (see GUIDELINES FOR HEALTHY EATING).
- If you are eating good food and committing your appetite to the Lord, but you still have cravings for the wrong foods and tend to overeat, then you may be exhibiting symptoms of a physical problem.
  - Seek the advice of a medical doctor. Your health is never

anything to take for granted or guess about.

- Obey the Bible's admonition to watch and pray so you don't enter into temptation; in other words, avoid tempting foods (Mark 14:38).
- When you find an emotional need that triggers binge eating, discover a non-food approach to satisfying your emotional need.[15]
- Keep busy doing something you enjoy, such as your work, a hobby, or something at which you are talented, such as singing.
- Bring every thought into captivity (II Corinthians 10:5).

TRY THESE PRACTICAL steps to help keep you from the temptation to overeat.

- Tell your family and friends that you have changed your diet and lifestyle.
  - You will be less inclined to go off your diet and will get extra support.
- Don't go in bakeries, doughnut shops, candy stores, and cookie shops.
- Train your eyes to rest only on healthful foods, not seductive sweets and meats that trigger binges.[16]
- Don't bring into your home the foods that tempt you to overeat—ice cream, cake, candy bars, doughnuts, cookies, etc.
  - When you have to buy for other family members, store the "forbidden fruit" in the back of your cupboard or refrigerator as soon as you get home.
- Always shop for foods *after* you have eaten.
  - Make a list and stick to it.
  - Take only enough money with you to pay for products on your list.
- When you eat, make that all you do.
  - Don't eat in the car, on the run, standing at the kitchen sink, or without thinking about what you are doing.

- Don't eat in front of the television set.
  - Don't watch television before you eat (the commercials are too tempting).[17]
- Eat a hearty breakfast.
  - Low blood sugar from fasting all night sinks even lower when you try to resist eating until noon.
  - In this weakened, half-starved state, you will be easily tempted by cravings and subject to binge eating.[18]
- Make eating a special occasion for the family or just for yourself—soft lights, attractive dishes and silverware, flowers, music, etc.
- Serve smaller portions.
  - Use smaller plates.
- Eat slowly and chew your food longer than you do now.
  - Chewing stimulates the flow of digestive juices.
  - When you take at least 20 minutes to eat, the message of a full stomach has the chance to reach your brain and turn off your desire to eat more.
- Don't leave the serving platter in front of you.
- Once you have finished eating, put the leftovers away.[19]
- Snack on carrot sticks or celery, a heaping tablespoon of cottage cheese, or a small apple.[20]

MANY OF US overeat occasionally and at certain times in our lives.

- In times of major change, extreme stress, disappointment, or illness, we will be tempted to overeat.
- If temptation should overcome you and you go on a binge, don't let it destroy your resolve to change your lifestyle.
  - Forgive yourself and start all over again.
  - It's better to continue striving than to give up.[21]

LEARN TO CONTROL yourself at restaurants and during the holidays.

- Search for restaurants with salad bars or that serve properly cooked vegetables and fresh fish, chicken, and meat.
  - Avoid restaurants that overcook their vegetables beyond

recognition.

- If the restaurant doesn't serve anything wholesome, just eat the best foods available.
- If you can't avoid a fast food restaurant or processed junk food, don't worry.
  - Eat a small dinner. If you are eating healthy foods on a regular basis and following God's principles for life, eating a fast-food dinner *once in a while* won't make that much of a difference.
- If you are invited to someone's house, go and be thankful for whatever they serve you.
  - Choose wisely at a buffet or potluck supper.
  - If you're not given a choice of foods, taste everything but don't go overboard.
- Don't feel guilty about having a piece of your birthday cake, chocolate mousse at your anniversary dinner, etc., but don't eat more than one piece.
- No matter the occasion, DO NOT GORGE.[22]

PRAY WITH ME, *"Father, in the name of Jesus, I commit my appetite to You. God, You've told me that the weight of my body and my attitude are hurting me, so I commit all of this into Your hands and ask You to be Lord of my appetite. Feed me with food that is convenient for me. In Jesus' name, Amen."*

THE BENEFITS OF EXERCISE

WHEN YOU'RE NOT keeping your mind or your body busy it becomes too easy to run to the refrigerator and help yourself to ice cream, leftovers, or tomorrow's lunch.

- Remaining idle will damage your body (Proverbs 27:7).
- Make a goal of doing moderate to vigorous exercise 30 to 60 minutes every day, or at least four to six times a week.

EXERCISE BENEFITS YOUR body in many ways.

- Exercise eliminates poisons, increases circulation, and

strengthens muscles.

■ Without exercise, impurities cannot be eliminated as they should, the blood does not circulate well, internal organs become inactive, and unused muscles shrink and weaken.[23]

- When you exercise you breathe deeply and inhale more oxygen.

  ■ Make sure to breathe deeply when exercising; you will do your body damage if you deny it oxygen when it needs it the most.

- Carbon dioxide and other poisons are removed from the body when you exhale.[24]

- Exercise strengthens the heart muscle.

  ■ The heart pumps more blood during exercise, sending all that extra oxygen you've just inhaled to the rest of your body.[25]

- Daily vigorous exercise is the best way to lower cholesterol.

  ■ It increases the ratio of good to bad cholesterol, and rids the blood of fats.[26]

- Exercise improves circulation.

  ■ When the blood does not circulate well, internal organs function at a bare minimum.[27]

- Exercise helps arteries and capillaries resist hardening.

  ■ Inactive capillaries often collapse and cannot provide enough food and oxygen to muscles and organs.[28]

- Exercise prevents and helps treat constipation.

  ■ It brings more blood, oxygen, and nutrients to the intestines to keep them toned up for easier and more efficient elimination of wastes.

- Prevention of hemorrhoids and relief from their symptoms can be accomplished with regular exercise.[29]

- Endorphins (chemicals in the brain that reduce pain and create a feeling of euphoria) are released during exercise.

  ■ Menstrual cramps and other painful problems are lessened

or eliminated with exercise because of endorphin release.
- Women with pre-menstrual syndrome (PMS) may find relief with regular exercise.[30]
- Daily exercise will help prevent, control, or even eliminate adult-onset diabetes.[31]
- Exercise may reduce or eliminate migraines.[32]
- Exercising with small to mid-sized weights can renew the strength of bones in older women (see NUTRITION VS. THE AGING PROCESS).
  - Exercise slows bone loss and bone softening.[33]
- Exercise improves your posture.
  - Weak muscles won't hold anything in place and lead to bad posture.
  - Bad posture leads to stooped shoulders, hunched back, hanging head, curvature of the spine, protruding stomach, and weak hips.
  - Bad posture causes frequent sprains, strains, pulls, pains, and dislocations.[34]
- Exercise increases your endurance.[35]
- Exercise develops muscle tissue.
  - The more muscle tissue you have, the higher your metabolism.
  - The higher your metabolism, the more calories you burn.
  - If you use more calories through exercise than you consume in food, you WILL lose fat.[36]
- Exercise will make you strong.
  - As you become stronger, you will feel more like getting out and doing things and being more active.
- Exercise relieves stress.
  - Tension and worries are greatly relieved by living an active life.[37]

SET ASIDE A specific time each day to exercise.
- Honor that time as you would any important appointment.
- Stay with it no matter what.[38]

CHOOSE AN ACTIVITY or group of activities.
- If you are out of shape and have not exercised for years, get clearance from your doctor for your new program.
- Choose something that will develop your entire body, not just one problem area.
- Buy books and magazines to make sure you are doing the exercises correctly and have the proper equipment.
  - Something as simple as wearing the wrong shoes can damage your leg muscles, bones, and knees.[39]
- If you are out of shape when you start your exercise program, you may be short of breath, weak, dizzy, nauseous, lightheaded, and tight chested.
  - If you experience these symptoms, lighten up on what you are doing.[40]
- Don't stop your exercise program if you are stiff or sore at the beginning.
  - You will eventually lose the aches and pains and replace those aggravations with energy, vigor, and strength.
  - If you stop exercising when you're sore and then start up again only to stop when you're sore again, you will never get through the sore stage.[41]
- If you get a sharp pain in your side when you exercise, you are probably holding your breath or breathing too shallowly.
  - A "stitch" occurs in your stomach muscles because waste builds in your body without enough oxygen.
  - It can also happen when you're out of shape or if you're exercising in hot and humid weather or in a place where there isn't enough ventilation.
- When you get a cramp of any kind, stop exercising and breathe slowly and deeply until it stops.[42]

AEROBIC EXERCISE IS rigorous and nonstop activity lasting 20 to 30 minutes.
- In addition to the standard aerobic classes, other aerobic activities are swimming, bicycling, jumping rope, jogging,

walking at a fast pace, or jumping on a mini-trampoline.[43]
IT'S NEVER TOO late to start.

- You can do all things through Christ Who strengthens you (Philippians 4:13).

TRY THESE EXERCISES at home.

- Start slowly.
- Gradually increase repetitions and difficulty.
- Be sure to breathe deeply. A way to test if you are not getting enough oxygen is to talk during your exercise (or count out loud).
  - ■ If you can't speak easily, you're working too hard too soon, which means you will tire faster, burn less fat, and negate the positive effects of exercise.

STRETCH—Stand and lean forward from the waist with your feet shoulder-width apart and your knees bent. Keep your back straight and your head down. Hold your hands behind your back with your elbows slightly bent. Slowly straighten your legs as you raise your clasped hands up and over your head. Hold for 10 to 30 seconds and slowly return to your original position. You will be stretching your arms, legs, and back. Don't bounce or lock your knees; only stretch gently until you feel the pull in your muscles.

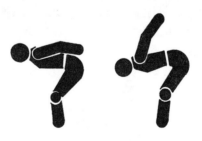

LUNGE—Stand tall with your chest up. Hold three-pound weights at your sides. Moving slowly, step forward with your right leg, making sure your front knee doesn't extend beyond your toe line, and keep your chest upright so your upper torso is perpendicular to your right thigh. Shift your weight to the front leg and straighten, lifting your back leg. Squeeze your buttocks and hold. Repeat, stepping forward with your left leg. Do two sets of 10 to 15 lunges with each leg.

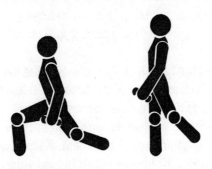

PULLING WEEDS—Stand with your knees bent and your right foot in front of your left leg. Put your right hand on a chair or low table. Hold onto 2- or 5-pound weights with your left hand and let your arm hang down. Pull the weight up to your armpit, making sure your elbow points to the ceiling and that your arm is close to your body. Slowly lower the weight and straighten your arm. Repeat 10 to 15 times. Work up to 8- to 10-pound weights.

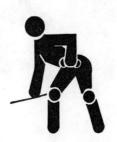

PUSH UPS—lie on your stomach on the bed and slide forward until you reach your hips (the more advanced you are, the farther down your body you can slide, until only your feet rest on the bed). Put your hands palm-down on the floor so they are directly below and slightly wider than your shoulders. Keep your back flat. Slowly bend your elbows and lower your chest to the floor (or as far as you can go); all the while tightening all your body's muscles. Straighten and repeat 10 to 15 times; do two sets.

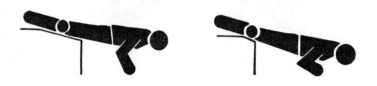

HANGING LAUNDRY—Crouch with your back parallel to the floor and your knees tucked into your chest. Hold 3- to 5-pound weights on the floor. In a smooth move, stand and curl the weights to your shoulders. Keep your stomach and buttock muscles tight and your knees slightly bent. Straighten your knees as you push the weights overhead. Reverse the moves and do two sets of 10 to 12 repetitions.

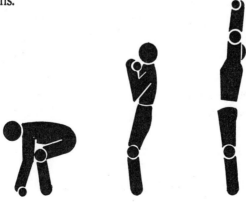

CRUNCH—Lie on your back with your hands behind your head, your knees bent, and your heels resting on a bed or in the air. Tighten your stomach muscles and lift your shoulders, pulling your knees to your chest. Reverse the move and do two sets of 10 to 15 repetitions.[44]

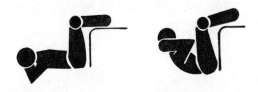

THE BENEFITS OF DRINKING WATER

WATER IS GOD'S perfect food (Proverbs 25:21).

- Water remains the same in your body.
- Your body's organs need water so they can perform well and keep you alive.
- Water carries blood corpuscles, nutrients, and wastes throughout your body.
- Water is continually passing away from the body, eliminating toxins and dead tissues through an organ of elimination, either your skin, kidneys, intestines, or lungs.
- Water dissolves poisons and separates them from body tissues.[45]

GOD DID NOT create soda pop, coffee, artificial fruit drinks, whiskey, or beer (Isaiah 44:3; II Peter 3:5).

- Carbonated drinks bloat you with gas.

- Sparkling mineral waters contain sodium.
- Coffee, tea, cocoa, and colas are dehydrating.
- Natural fruit juices contain water and are very good for you; but they are a food, and the body must process them differently.[46]

DRINK 64 OUNCES (eight 8-ounce glasses) of fresh, pure water every day.

- If you are overweight, live in an arid area, do hard labor, exercise, run, or do other dehydrating tasks, you need to drink more than 64 ounces of water a day.
- Drink 16 ounces 30-45 minutes before breakfast, lunch, supper, and bedtime.
  - Do not drink these 16 ounces of water less than one half hour before meals or within two hours after you eat.
  - You don't need to drink with meals (a couple of sips is fine) because the extra liquid will weaken your digestive juices.
- NEVER substitute anything for water.[47]

IF YOU HAVE trouble swallowing water, put a few drops of lemon or orange juice in the water to make it palatable.

- If you experience difficulty drinking water, mix half water and half juice and gradually diminish the amount of juice over time.[48]

WATER THAT CONTAINS more impurities than you do won't cleanse your system.

- God will provide you good water when you are in need (Isaiah 41:17).
- Drink bottled water if your public water supply contains germs, algae, and parasites and is treated with an abundance of chemicals or your well water is contaminated with heavy metals or harmful bacteria.
  - NOTE: If you develop sores in your mouth after drinking tap water you may be allergic or sensitive to the chemicals used for water treatment, so buy bottled water.

- If you drink purified or distilled water, eat foods high in minerals in order to replace the minerals you are not getting in your drinking water.[49]

SANCTIFY YOUR FOOD

TO SANCTIFY YOUR FOOD means to set it apart with prayer.

- When you set your food apart by praying over it, God said He would make it special for you (I Timothy 4:3-5).
- When you pray over your food, God's blessings come upon that food and it benefits your health.

WHEN YOU HAVE situations in which you don't have proper foods because you are poor or you are in some area where proper food is not available, God will put proper nutrition in your food when you sanctify it through prayer.

- I've had times when I know what I've eaten could have been very upsetting to my system, but I've prayed and asked God to protect me by blessing that food and sanctifying it.
- I've been all over the world, eaten in all kinds of situations and circumstances, and I have not been sick.
  - ■ I have been healthy because I believe my food is sanctified by the Word of God and prayer (I Timothy 4:5).

WHEN YOU PRAY over your food, say, "God, I believe this food is so nutritious and healthy, and You are taking away anything in it that will hurt me."

- If you need help with your appetite or what you eat, bless your food.
- God will sanctify it and take sickness away from it (Deuteronomy 7:13-15).

SOME CHRISTIANS GET flaky with this and say, "That makes it all right for me to eat a whole pecan pie."

- Don't turn off your brain and think that sanctifying your food works even when you act like an idiot.
- Don't ask God to bless junk food so you can fulfill your bad appetite.

- If you break natural laws, God won't bless you.
  - If you go to the top of a building and say, "I'm going to jump off and angels will catch me," you're going to break your neck because you are breaking the laws of gravity.

THE KINGDOM OF FOOD

LOOK AT EVERYTHING you do. Do you glorify the Lord in what you say, eat, and do (I Corinthians 10:31)?
- Keep the right attitude.
- Read the Bible.
- Pray.

THE KINGDOM OF God is not meat and drink. It is righteousness, peace, and joy in the Holy Ghost (Romans 14:17).
- Do not dwell on your eating habits, or on whether you are too fat or too skinny.
- Take your eyes off the problem, and put your eyes on the kingdom of God.
- Understand that your body belongs to the Lord.
- Make eating a spiritual event, as it was meant to be.

IF YOUR EATING is put in the proper place, as a part of God's kingdom, then you will do it with peace and joy and you will be healthy (Acts 27:34).
- You will receive life and resurrection power from your food, rather than death and corruption.

TAKE THE RESURRECTION power that Jesus gave you in the communion service and treat all your meals the same way.
- Celebrate that not only did you die in Christ, but you are also raised in Christ.
- If you eat as if it were communion with the Lord, then when you face crisis situations, food will have resurrection power for you.
- You are not eating just to get by. You eat in order to receive life and to have it more abundantly.

73

WINNING OVER THE WEIGHTS OF LIFE

Your attitude toward yourself and others affects your health. It's not just what you eat that determines whether you're healthy or sick, but also the inward attitudes or "weights" that you allow to take up residence in your heart.

Man is a three-fold being—spirit, soul, and body (I Thessalonians 5:23). To be a complete, content person, the needs of all three parts have to be met. Your physical needs can be met— getting enough rest, eating the right foods—but you can be a basket case mentally and emotionally.

Proverbs 20:27 says, *"The spirit of man is the candle of the LORD, searching all the inward parts of the belly."* Your spirit man is where God can bring new life. By His Spirit He will show you where you are out of sync, and He will cause life to flow into your physical body.

What is in your heart—envy, anger, bitterness, all manner of evil, cruelty, fear, depression, immorality—affects your spirit, soul, and body. If you harbor anything in your heart that's contrary to the Word of God, it will eventually begin to eat away at you physically.

The root cause of most sickness and disease can be directly related to the attitudes of the heart. If you can get your attitudes in line with the Word of God, you can totally turn your health situation around.

YOUR HEART AND THE INNER MAN

YOUR HEART HAS to do with your inner man.

- There are 821 references in the Bible to a man's heart; they refer primarily to the inner or spirit man.

THE HEART IS like a computer that has volumes of information stored in its memory bank.

- Keep your heart clear of extraneous material so it functions as God created it.
  - Cleanse your heart of wrong attitudes and wrong thinking (I John 1:9).
  - *"Keep thy heart with all diligence; for out of it are the issues of life"* (Proverbs 4:23).

SOMETIMES WE BLAME external things for the lack of good health, when the real issue is the attitude of our hearts (see SHEDDING THE HABITS THAT WEIGH YOU DOWN).

- Even the Biblical characters who got into trouble (i.e., Saul), had inner problems (like jealousy) that manifested in the natural realm.
- Blaming the devil won't maintain or restore your health.
  - Blaming the devil only diverts your attention from the "root" cause of the problem.
  - The devil takes advantage of everything he can, but he's not the cause of every traumatic situation.
  - The "root" cause can be found by examining the attitudes of your heart.

THE IMPORTANCE OF ATTITUDES AND YOUR BONES

WRONG ATTITUDES ARE harmful because they can defeat you spiritually.

- Attitudes that cause anxiety and depression are often related to family problems, unhappy work situations, and the wrong attitude toward yourself and others.
- Good attitudes are like medicine to your bones and health to all your flesh.

BONES ARE THE very foundation of your body, and have to do with health and life.

- In the past, bones were thought to be very stable, unchanging tissues, but we now know that metabolically they are changing daily.

- Your blood cells are made in the bone marrow, so your health is determined by what is in your bones.
- If the marrow tissue of bone is diseased, then the entire composition of blood is affected.
  - We can then conclude that life is in the bones, as well as in the blood.
- The health of your bones is determined by your attitude.
  - Attitudes such as fear, anxiety, depression, and resentment can be manifested physically.
  - Researchers say resentment and bitterness are two of the most common attitudes that affect health.
  - Many physical and emotional problems today are caused by depression and anxiety.
  - Stress can affect your hormone level, heart rate, blood pressure, and certain elements in the blood.
  - The secretions of the stomach, the digestive tract, and the contractions of the digestive tract are actually changed by certain levels of stress.

GOD PUTS A lot of importance on bones because the health of the flesh is in the bones.

- When Adam saw Eve he was delighted, and said she is "... *now bone of my bones, and flesh of my flesh:* ... " (Genesis 2:23).
- The Israelites carried Joesph's bones out of Egypt when they left (Genesis 50:25; Exodus 13:19).

AS THE BRIDE of Christ, we are bone of His bone, and flesh of His flesh. Ephesians 5:30 says "... *we are members of his body, of his flesh, and of his bones."*

- Not a bone of Jesus' body was broken.
- The prayer of Jesus was that we be one, not one bone broken; not one member out of place.
- Bones are highly significant in the creation of God (see

SHEDDING THE HABITS THAT WEIGH YOU DOWN).
ADULTERY CAN DESTROY the physical body.

- The wounds and hurts perpetrated by marital infidelity can literally cause your bones to rot.
- *"A virtuous woman is a crown to her husband: but she that maketh ashamed is as rottenness in his bones"* (Proverbs 12:4).

ENVY AFFECTS THE structure of your bones.

- *"A sound heart is the life of the flesh: but envy the rottenness of the bones"* (Proverbs 14:30).
- Blood cells are made in the bone marrow.
  - Envy affects your blood and poisons your health.
  - Many people are sick today and have blood diseases and other problems because of envy.

SAUL'S JEALOUSY of David caused him to lose his anointing, backslide, and commit suicide (I Samuel 16,28,31).

- Jealousy opens the door for evil spirits to attack your mind, will, and emotions.
- Allowing envy to continue in your life opens the door to a host of physical ailments.

LONGEVITY AND YOUR HEART

YOUR HEART ATTITUDE determines how long (and healthily) you will live.

- *"My son, forget not my law; but let thine heart keep my commandments: For length of days, and long life, and peace, shall they add to thee"* (Proverbs 3:1,2).
- God created man to obey Him.
- Disobedience to the Word causes man to get off balance, which affects every level of life (Proverbs 9:11; 10:27).

LONGEVITY IS A result of more than just plenty of exercise, rest, and the proper diet.

- A heart full of bitterness, anger, unforgiveness, and sin will

shorten your life span.
- Your heart attitude today determines tomorrow's health.

THE TRIPLETS

BITTERNESS, STRIFE, AND confusion are triplets. Strife breeds confusion; confusion breeds bitterness.
- Bitterness is a "taste" as well as an attitude.
- Bitterness can hinder your prayer life.
- Bitterness can defile you (Hebrews 12:15).
- Esau became bitter when his brother, Jacob, stole his blessing (Genesis 27).
- Bitterness is contagious.
- Esau's bitterness caused a family curse on his future generations.
  - Esau's descendants, the Edomites, were bitter against Jacob's descendants (Numbers 20:14-21).

FORGIVENESS, AN ACT OF VIOLENCE

UNFORGIVENESS CAUSES BITTERNESS (see SHEDDING THE HABITS THAT WEIGH YOU DOWN).
- Unforgiveness is a heavy-duty weight.
  - It can affect your thinking, strength, anointing, health, and the direction of your life.
  - Unforgiveness creates a chemical imbalance, and causes sickness and disease in your bones (Proverbs 15:30; 17:22).

FORGIVENESS IS AN act of violence.
- Forgiveness paralyzes the hand of the devil.
- It "sends away" the incident (Ephesians 4:26,27).
- God forgives by removing our transgressions from us

(Psalms 103:12).
- Forgiveness is not weakness but an aggressive force.
- Through forgiveness you are protected from the evil acts of men and Satan.
- When you harbor unforgiveness in your heart, you give place to the devil to wreak havoc in your life and your physical body.
  - Unforgiveness brings death to your life by causing you to focus on the person who committed the offense.
  - Forgiveness takes the sting out of the offense and causes you to focus on Jesus.

FORGIVENESS FOSTERS CHANGE.
- It releases you and the person who has offended you from the offense.
- It frees God to bring about a change in both of you.
- The power of your redemption was released on the Cross.

THERE ARE FOUR steps to forgiving.
1) Understand that the devil is responsible for the offense.
2) Separate the person from the sin.
   - Hate the sin, not the person.
   - Get mad at the devil.
3) Make the decision NOW to forgive everyone who has ever offended you.
4) Bless those who have offended you according to Luke 6:27,28.

UNFORGIVENESS CAUSES DEPRESSION.
- Don't take depression lightly.
- It can decay your bones (Psalms 31:10).
- *"A merry heart doeth good like a medicine: but a broken spirit drieth the bones"* (Proverbs 17:22).

DEPRESSION IS MORE THAN JUST AN ATTITUDE

DEPRESSION IS A sickness treatable with medication.
- Fear is the opposite of faith, and fear can lead to depression.
- Anything that's not of faith is sin (see SHEDDING THE HABITS THAT WEIGH YOU DOWN).
- It deals with both the spirit and soul of man.
  - Depression starts in the spirit man and affects the soul of man.
  - Depression causes you to feel burdened, gloomy, and sad.
  - Depression is an open door to the devil's attacks.

THE ROOT OF most depression is disobedience and rebellion against God.
- Saul was a good king until he rebelled against God (I Samuel 13 and 15).
- Saul became depressed because he lost his kingdom and evil spirits began to vex him (I Samuel 16).
  - David was summoned to play for Saul because music seemed to soothe him.
- Depression created a mental imbalance in Saul.
  - His depression gave way to jealousy and an obsession to kill David (I Samuel 19).

BAD CIRCUMSTANCES CAN also cause depression.
- Tamar was heavy in spirit because her father-in-law broke his promise to her (see Genesis 38).
- David yielded to depression after his adulterous involvement with Bath-sheba (see II Samuel 11,12).

DON'T EAT WHEN you are depressed.
- If you eat only when you are happy, it will be a feast to you.
  - *"All the days of the afflicted are evil: but he that is of a merry heart **hath a continual feast**"* (Proverbs 15:15).
- If you are depressed or emotionally distraught, your food

will knot up in your stomach.
- ■ Eating at times like these can cause ulcers and other physical illnesses.
- ■ People get ulcers by eating when they have unforgiveness and hatred in their hearts.
- ■ Correct your attitude and then eat with joy. You will have a continual feast.
  - • You will receive more strength from your food if you eat it with joy (Nehemiah 8:10).

FIGHT DEPRESSION WITH joy.
- • Sing songs, hymns, and spiritual songs unto the Lord.
- • Cast your depression on the Lord, and begin to sing and worship Him.

NOT ALL FAT IS BAD

"FAT" IS NOT popular in today's society.
- • "Fat" in the Bible has to do with God's anointing (Proverbs 15:30).
- • The anointing breaks yokes, improves your mind and emotions, and saturates your bones.
- • When a dead man's body was thrown on top of Elisha's bones, the bones held such an anointing that the dead man was resurrected (II Kings 13:20,21).

A GOOD REPORT brings an anointing to your bones. Bad reports can take away your health.
- • Gossip and talebearing affect your anointing and health.
- • *"The north wind driveth away rain: so doth an angry countenance a backbiting tongue"* (Proverbs 25:23).

A SOFT TONGUE breaks the bones of contention, and brings health to your bones (Proverbs 15:1).
- • *"Pleasant words are as an honeycomb, sweet to the soul, and health to the bones"* (Proverbs 16:24).

CRUELTY WILL TROUBLE your own flesh.

- No one can get away with being cruel to others.
- Scripture says if you are cruel to others your own flesh will eventually fight against you (Proverbs 11:17).
  - Show mercy to others and you'll help your mind and emotions.
- Regardless of what others have done to you, you have to forgive them with the forgiveness of Jesus.
  - Surrender all bitterness and cruelty to Him.
  - Show cruelty to people and you'll cause your own flesh to become sick.

THE DOWNSIDE OF FEAR

FEAR AFFECTS MORE than your faith.

- Fear adversely affects your mind, body, and emotions (see SHEDDING THE HABITS THAT WEIGH YOU DOWN).
- *"Fear came upon me, and trembling, which made all my bones to shake"* (Job 4:14).
  - Doctors say fear can affect the body to the point of causing sickness, cancer, and other diseases.
  - Fear caused Job to become so skinny and sick that his bones and flesh became one, as though they were glued together. (See Job 19:20.)

FEAR IS BONDAGE.

- Once a fear is entertained in your mind it can grow and become a stronghold.
- Fear can cause your thinking to become unstable.
  - Fear has torment (I John 4:18).

PUTTING YOUR FAITH in circumstances instead of in the Bible is the root cause of fear.

- Peter walked on water, but when he saw "... *the wind boisterous, he was afraid; and* [began] *to sink,...* " (Matthew 14:30).

THE FEAR OF the Lord will keep you walking in the same

direction (Proverbs 1:7).

A HEART FIXED on the Lord can protect you from fear (Psalms 112:7).

- Faith in the Word can fix and stabilize your heart and cause you to be "fear free."
- You don't have to remain fearful.
  - Resist fear (II Timothy 1:7; James 4:7).

THE JOY OF THE LORD

LAUGHING CAN MAKE you well.

- Medical research has proven that people who laugh a lot have fewer heart attacks.
- Eating is very much a laughing matter.
- Laughter has to do with your attitude, your health, and with the way you are received by others (Proverbs 17:22).

GOD MEETS PEOPLE who laugh or rejoice in Him (Isaiah 64:5).

- Rejoicing in the Lord elevates you above the situation and enables you to enter into a childlike faith.
  - Laughing allows God to move quickly and freely to turn your circumstances around.

LAUGH AT DISASTER because you've already won (Job 5:22; I Corinthians 15:57).

- The Bible says bad circumstances are temporary, but the Word of God will last forever.
- Continue to rejoice in the Lord until you see a breakthrough in your situation (Philippians 4:4; Hebrews 3:6).

SELF-PITY IS a party no one wants to be invited to but you.

- It causes you to take your eyes off the supernatural.
- You yield to self-pity when you begin to think and talk about the problem.
  - This sets the stage for the devil to steal your joy.
  - When your joy leaves, so does your strength and your body's ability to fight off disease (Nehemiah 8:10).

LAUGHING IMPROVES YOUR appearance.
- A merry countenance makes you attractive.
  - *"A merry heart maketh a cheerful countenance: but by the sorrow of the heart the spirit is broken"* (Proverbs 15:13).
- You could spend millions of dollars on your outward appearance; but if you have a sad countenance, you are unattractive to others.

IT'S DANGEROUS NOT to be joyful.
- Joyfully thank God for what He's done, or you could lose what you have (Deuteronomy 28:47,48).

A LAUGH A day keeps the devil away.
- God laughs at the devil, and we should join Him in the fun.
- *"The Lord shall laugh at him: for he seeth that his day is coming"* (Psalms 37:13).
- Onions and circumstances can make you cry; the Word of God can make you laugh.
- Rejoicing is important because God is in the midst of your praises (Psalms 22:3).
- Rejoicing communicates to the devil that you have already won (I Corinthians 15:57).

MAKE A DECISION to rejoice in every situation instead of waiting for the circumstances to dictate how you feel.
- Don't allow the circumstance to determine your spiritual state.
- Take control of every situation with praise and worship.

PAUL AND SILAS opened prison doors by rejoicing in the midst of what looked like an impossible situation (Acts 16:25-34).
- Paul and Silas set an atmosphere of joy instead of letting the atmosphere set their mood.
- God met them in prison, in the midst of their praises.
  - In the midst of their praises, there was an earthquake that opened the doors of the prison.

SWEET SLEEP

CHRISTIANS ARE PROMISED "sweet sleep." If you consistently experience sleepless nights, the devil is robbing you of something God guarantees (Proverbs 3:21-24).

- Sleepless nights can be a sign of eating the wrong thing, or a fearful, angry, or fretful attitude.
- Memorize Scriptures, meditate on the Word during those sleepless periods, and cast all of your care on God.
- When you meditate on God's Word, the Word will lead you, keep you, and speak to you during your waking and sleeping moments (Proverbs 6:22).
  - Let God's Word cleanse your heart of all unrighteousness (Ephesians 5:26).

SHEDDING THE HABITS THAT WEIGH YOU DOWN

YOUR HEART AND THE ISSUES OF LIFE

YOU MUST TAKE care of your heart because out of it come the issues of life.

- Your *heart* is your "spirit," which is the hidden man of the Lord (I Peter 3:4).
  - Your heart will not corrupt.
- The issues of your life will either be health, prosperity, happiness, peace, and joy; or they will be sin, bad attitudes, hatefulness, sadness, despair, and death.

ALTHOUGH YOUR HEART is not corruptible, your soul (mind and emotions) are, which will cause you trouble.

- If you allow your soul to rule over your life, you will create bad habits that can cause physical destruction or early death.
  - Habits are created through a process that begins with a single thought.
  - Dwelling on certain thoughts can lead to actions.
  - When the actions continue, they become habits.
  - Through habits you reap a lifestyle, and that can either bring death or abundant life.
    - * When you allow God to guide your spirit, He will control your mind and emotions and give you life more abundantly (John 10:10).

YOU NEED REGULAR heart checkups (I'm not talking about a physical exam) so the Holy Spirit can check for bitterness, fearfulness, depression, or hatefulness.

- Ask God to tell you if there is any wicked way in you.
- When you listen for the truth about your heart, He can deal with you effectively.
- Repent of your negative emotions.
- God will strengthen your soul and give you a steadfast heart so you can be victorious in your situations and circumstances (Psalms 138:3).

KEEP A RIGHT attitude in the various changes of your life, hold onto God, and say what the Word says—you'll come through very well.

- Spend time in the Word.
- Spend time in prayer.
- Keep your confidence and faith in God.

A WOUNDED ATTITUDE AND YOUR HEART

YOUR HEART CAN'T be wounded by outside forces. What breaks your heart is **your own attitude.**

- A wounded attitude (or an attitude of bitterness) will hurt your spirit and body.
  - When I eat something bitter, my mouth contracts like it's in pain and my teeth are set on edge.
  - A bitter attitude (being angry, discontented) sets your physical body on edge.
- You can become bitter if you don't forgive and forget the hurts that are heaped on you by your spouse, children, mother, father, employers, neighbors, and government.
  - You may feel you have a right to be bitter because of your pain, but that bitterness will hurt you more than the other people's actions.

THE ROOT OF bitterness grows a variety of fruit, including hatefulness, self-loathing, despair, strife, jealousy, and confusion.

- That bitter fruit is shared with others, and when they taste

your fruit, they can become bitter too.
- ■ When you spread your bitterness to others, YOU will be defiled.
- • I believe bitterness hinders your faith.
  - ■ When you harbor a wounded attitude, you aren't trusting God to take care of you, heal you, and avenge you.
  - ■ Lack of faith keeps God from hearing your prayers.

WHEN YOU FEEL bitter, examine the reason you feel the way you do and get rid of it by laying it at Jesus' feet (Ephesians 4:31).
- • Job was angry and discontented (Job 7:11; 10:1).
  - ■ Job was weary of life.
  - ■ He was full of complaints and accusations against God.
  - ■ Job was set free of his bitterness when he repented (Job 42:6).
    - * God turned Job's situation around and gave Job a double portion of what he had before his trials.
- • When you repent, God will forgive and cleanse you (Psalms 50:15; I John 1:9).
  - ■ When Jesus died on the Cross, he drank the bitter cup of our sins.
  - ■ Our bitterness will be cleansed by the blood of Jesus.
- • If you don't repent of the sin of bitterness, you will keep it and it will grow.

BITTERNESS CAN BE used positively.
- • A bitter circumstance can cause you to reach out to God, to repent, and to recommit your life to Him.
  - ■ Jeremiah was bitter over the destruction of Judah and Jerusalem.
    - * He wept in a bitterness of the soul because the people were taken into captivity; the women were raped and killed; the children were killed; and the young men were led away as slaves to Babylon.
    - * I believe God let Jeremiah feel what He Himself felt for His people.

- In Jeremiah's case, bitterness was a bad taste, but it wasn't a bad attitude.
    * Jeremiah's bitterness was grief.
- If you don't allow grief to follow its natural course (you must allow yourself to feel the pain and you must take it to the Lord), you will become angry and discontented.
    * When you feel bitter, turn to God so He can move in the situation and heal your attitude.

GOSSIP AND YOUR HEART

SOMETIMES WE ACT like gossip is harmless, frivolous, and meaningless. But God doesn't consider gossip harmless—He has some very strong things to say about talebearers, slanderers, and scorners!

- Leviticus 19:16 tells us we should NOT gossip under any circumstances.

PEOPLE WHO GOSSIP have some very ugly traits.

- People who gossip want to be accepted by their peers, but aren't willing to be anyone's true friend.
    - They say, "If I have some gossip, people will listen to me. They'll think I have something to say."
    - Their motives are to tear down someone else so they will be uplifted.
- A gossip tells everyone your strictest confidences and meddles in other people's affairs.
    - Proverbs 11:13 says, *"A talebearer revealeth secrets: but he that is of a faithful spirit concealeth the matter."*
    - A person who has a faithful spirit would never tell anyone's secrets. That person is a witness to the way God treats His children.
- People who gossip are critical and scornful (Proverbs 1:22).
    - They tell you what's wrong with every ministry, every person, every marriage, every child, everything.

90

> * They tell you what the problem is, but they never offer a solution.
> - They always put something down, saying they can do it much better.
>> * They always say they know more than anyone else.
>> * They are experts with no practice.

- People who gossip are proud and don't want anyone to tell them what is wrong with their own lives; in other words, they don't like to be judged (Proverbs 19:28).
  - They will attack someone if they are corrected.
    * They always say their problems are caused by someone else.
  - They don't submit to God.
    * They won't allow judgment to come on their sin because they won't search their hearts.
- People who gossip don't have enough to do (Psalm 123:4).
- People who gossip are fools (Proverbs 10:18).
  - A *fool* is someone who "believes God doesn't exist."
    * Gossips don't believe God is always with them, that He cares about their attitudes and actions, or that His Word is the truth.

IF YOU GOSSIP, you are on God's abomination list and you will bring suffering to yourself and to others.

- A person who gossips causes the same pain as a murderer, a thief, and an evildoer (I Peter 4:15).
- When you gossip, other people will gossip about you, but the information can be twice as damaging (Galatians 5:15).
- When you gossip, your children pick up the habit and make it their own.
  - They will suffer the effects of your sin and their own sin of gossiping (Exodus 20:5).

TO GET SET free from gossiping, realize that this is a heavy-duty sin and must not be treated lightly.

- Repent.

- Ask God for His help so you never do it again.
    - If you are concerned about someone and want to discuss the particulars of that person's situation with someone else—*that is gossiping*, no matter how heart-felt your reasons may be.
    - Take your concerns to God in prayer.
- Turn your attention to God.

GOD DOES NOT want talebearing to continue, so when you are led by the Holy Spirit to deal with a gossip, you have several ways to handle the problem.

- Proverbs 20:19 tells you to steer clear of talebearers.
    - Every now and then somebody will come to me with what they consider to be really "juicy" information. Although I want people to like me, I want to please God more. So, I say, "This conversation is not comfortable to me. I feel uncomfortable having you talk to me about this. Can we talk about something else?"
        * If that person doesn't appreciate what I've said lovingly, he will not return.
- Proverbs 19:25 says you should *"smite a scorner, ..."*
    - Although I don't recommend you slap people around, you can hit them hard with loving, corrective words.
- If the Holy Spirit leads you to confront a gossip (I call confronting someone "CAREfronting"), do it!
- Say it in a loving attitude.
- Everything you say must come from the Lord (from His Word and your heart).
    - One time at our church, a couple who came as guest speakers started talking terribly against another ministry and the pastors with whom they had just worked. I knew that when they left us, they would say the same kind of things about my husband and me. I thought, "Oh, God, that's terrible. They're young converts and they're getting into a lot of trouble."

- ■ The Lord told me to write them and "CAREfront" them. After I prayed about what I was going to write, I told them honestly what they had done and why it was wrong scripturally.
- ■ When they responded, they were so sweet and wonderful. They wrote back and said, "You are exactly right. The instant we got on the plane, we started talking about what we saw was your weakness and where we thought you were blowing it. This is a terrible thing in our lives, and we appreciate you being direct and honest."
- • If you are still not getting through to the gossiper, Proverbs 22:10 says, *"Cast out the scorner, and contention shall go out; yea, strife and reproach shall cease."*
  - ■ You will usually find the root of strife and confusion in a work or church situation to be gossip.

FEAR AND YOUR HEART

WHAT ARE YOU afraid of? Do you fear the dark, your parents, losing your home, being audited by the I.R.S., getting fired? That kind of fear will do nothing but raise your blood pressure and kill your hope. But the fear of God will give you wisdom and great blessings.

- • Proverbs 28:14 tells us that a person who fears the Lord is a happy person, but a person who thinks God won't punish him or chastise him will get into trouble.
  - ■ You will be happy when you learn to fear God by holding Him in reverence and dreading the wrath of His anger.
- • Proverbs 15:16 says, *"Better is little with the fear of the LORD than great treasure and trouble therewith."*
  - ■ The Lord will help you walk in the right direction because He gives you guidelines for living a safe, happy, and healthy life.

      * Just as your parents told you to keep your fingers away from fire, God's Word shows you how to be safe and not get burned by the devil.

- We should revere what His Word says because if God said it, He meant it!

YOU GET INTO trouble with fear when it is directed toward situations and other people. That kind of fear is filled with dread and devoid of faith.

- Fear starts in your life when you look at your circumstances instead of Jesus.
  - When Jesus walked on the water, Peter asked if he could join Him (Matthew 14:25-30).
    * Wanting to follow Jesus was an act of faith.
  - When Peter looked at the winds and the waves, he began to sink.
    * Peter almost drowned because he took his eyes off Jesus.
- Fear of circumstances will torment your spirit and your body.
  - The spirit of fear will move in all areas of your life, hindering and hurting you.
  - Fear will cause physical problems (Job 4:14, 19:20; Habakkuk 3:16).
- Once you give in to your fears, they will grow and grow until they become bondages.
  - Fear is contagious.
    * Your fears can be fed by other people, news reports, and coincidences.
- Fear can make you unstable in your thinking.
  - When you let it go for too long, fear becomes a phobia which will envelop your mind and hold you tight in paranoia (Proverbs 28:1).

GOD WILL RELEASE you from your fear.

- Fix your heart on the Word of God (Psalms 112:7).
  - His Word will stabilize your emotions and fix your heart

on God.
- The more you have the Word and the more you hold onto it, the more established you are in His promises and blessings.
    * You have His miracle-working power in your life.
    * You have His love (John 3:16).
    * You have the mind of Christ (I Corinthians 2:16).
    * You have His protection (Psalms 23:4; Proverbs 1:33).
- Believe God can take all things and work them together for good (Romans 8:28).
    - When you are afraid, talk to God and tell Him, "Lord, I'm going to trust You to take care of me in this matter."
- Saturate yourself in God's love.
    - God's perfect love casts out all fear.

GOD LOVES AND cares for you and wants to take away your fears (II Timothy 1:7).
- He will deliver you (Psalms 34:4).
    - When Peter sank in the water, Jesus rescued him (Matthew 14:31,32).
        * Jesus didn't leave him there and say, "Well, Buddy, you're in fear, not in faith. So, sink away."
    - Jesus wants to deliver you from your fears and encourage you in your faith.
        * The disciples were afraid after Christ's death that they would be crucified too, so they hid behind locked doors.
        * When Jesus came and stood in the midst of them He said, "Peace be unto you"; not "Hey, why didn't you guys trust Me and believe what I told you?"
    - Jesus offers us peace, not condemnation.
- When you are afraid, be honest with the Lord (Psalms 34:4).
    - Tell Him that you are afraid, that you don't like it, you feel it's the opposite of faith, you're sorry for it, and you repent of it (Psalms 56:3).

DEPRESSION AND YOUR HEART

DEPRESSION IS CAUSED by several things—lack of faith, difficult situations, or a chemical imbalance in your body.

- Depression is a horrible weight on your heart.
- Depression makes a way for the enemy to come in and attack you.
- When you are depressed you will say things that are not true about yourself and other people.
- When you are depressed, you will do things you would not normally do because you are allowing the darkness of your emotions to reign over you, rather than letting God heal you.
- Depression can lead people to suicide.

SOME DEPRESSION IS caused by disobedience and rebellion against God.

- King Saul is a classic case of depression in the Bible, but he didn't start out being depressed.
  - When Samuel anointed him as king, Saul was a fine young man and a good ruler.
  - When he got into rebellion against God, his problems started.
- Saul was jealous of David and became bitter, hateful, and depressed.
- Saul's jealousy became an obsession to kill David.
- His obsession opened the door for evil spirits to possess him.
  - Depression opens the door for evil spirits to come against your mind, emotions, and physical body.
- His attitude and situations got so bad that, in desperation, he sought the counsel of a witch.
- Saul's depression led to his suicide during battle.
- Like Saul, many Christians who rebel against God in any area of their lives (eating, exercising, reading the Bible, prayer,

witnessing, maintaining a godly lifestyle, etc.) are opening the window of their hearts for depression to enter instead of opening the door for Jesus to come in.

■ The devil will get into your heart through the open window of depression.

• Repent of your disobedience or rebellion and you will be set free.

■ If Saul would have turned to the Word of God and done what the Word said, obeyed the Word, and spoken the Word, he would not have become a broken and decayed man.

■ He didn't see a way out because he didn't look to God for his relief.

SELF-PITY CAN bring on depression.

• When you start thinking about your situation, you dwell on it.

• Then you start to talk about it.

■ When you tell one person about your problems, you think, "This situation is worse than I thought."

■ Then you tell someone else and you think, "This is the pits. I'm not going to make it."

* When you talk with an attitude of self-pity, you build yourself a coffin of despair.

• People who say they are "burned-out" at work, in a relationship, or in church are involved in self-pity.

• You set the stage for the devil when you get into self-pity.

■ When you say, "I can't take it anymore," the devil takes over.

* He will walk right into your life and say, "That's right, you can't take it anymore. Let's steal from you what God has given you." And he'll walk away with it.

• Self-pity robs you of joy.

■ When your joy leaves, your strength leaves.

* Groaning in self-pity will cause physical problems (Psalms 102:5).

- Speak positive words about your life.
  - Your inner man hears everything you say and he will bring to pass what you say.
  - When you are joyful in your situations, your inner man hears that and begins to rejoice.
  - Set your atmosphere, don't let the atmosphere set you!

YOU CAN TAKE steps to get out of these types of depression.

- Repent of rebellion, lack of faith, lying, hatred, etc.
  - David got involved in a wounded spirit and a depressed attitude because he didn't repent of his adultery with Bathsheba and the murder of her husband.
    * When Nathan confronted David, David repented.
    * God forgave David after he repented.
    * David's life turned around, his depression lifted, and he entered back into the joy of the Lord.
- When you confess your sins, God is faithful and just to forgive your sins and cleanse you from all unrighteousness (I John 1:9).

SOMETIMES DEPRESSION COMES on us after a loss or a desperate situation.

- When you experience the painful emotions of grief or loss, don't push them below the surface.
  - If you feel pain, cry!
    * Even if it wouldn't be appropriate or if you are afraid to open the floodgates, crying will keep your heart from becoming dull.
- God wants you to openly acknowledge your feelings (Ecclesiastes 3:1,4)
  - Go to the Lord with your tears so He can heal you.
- You must learn to go through all the stages of grief. You must allow yourself to mourn the loss of a dream, your childhood, a part of your body, a marriage, a loved one, etc.
  - Don't shut off your feelings of loss because you are cheating yourself of a complete healing.

- ■ Listen to what you are feeling and ask God to help you identify and deal with it.[1]
- Don't avoid grief out of fear.
  - ■ You won't be consumed by your grief because God will give you release.
- Your emotions should not rule your life, nor should you make decisions based on them; but you shouldn't ignore them either.[2]
- Even when you feel pain, rejoice in the Lord (Hebrews 3:6).
  - ■ When you stay joyful in Him, you are showing Him that you trust Him to carry you through the pain.
- Remember that the circumstances and your pain won't last forever (Psalms 30:5).
  - ■ Joy is coming, so hold onto God's promises and try not to lose your faith.
- It is dangerous not to be joyful (Deuteronomy 28:47,48).
  - ■ If you don't stay joyful and thank God for what He has done, joy, gladness of heart, and abundance of all things can leave you forever.
  - ■ When you spend your life grieving, your physical health will deteriorate (Psalms 31:10; Proverbs 17:22).
- Laugh at the devil in the face of disaster (Job 5:22).
  - ■ That's exactly what Paul and Silas did.
    - * They had been beaten and thrown in prison.
    - * At midnight they weren't cursing God over their situation, they were rejoicing in the Lord.

DEEP, CHRONIC DEPRESSION, according to the U.S. Public Health Service, is a physical problem that affects about 11 million people in the United States yearly.[3]

- It is a malfunction of the chemicals in your body that affects your mental health as well as your physical health.
- Medical and psychological evidence says the cause of chronic depression may be an unbalanced interaction of chemicals in the brain, the pituitary gland (an organ in the brain that

influences growth, metabolism, and maturation), and the kidneys.[4]

- Depression cost the United States about $27 billion in medical care, worker absenteeism, and other costs in 1989 alone.[5]
- The U.S. Public Health Service said chronic depression can generally be diagnosed by the following symptoms, which must be present all day, every day, for at least two weeks:
  - Depressed mood
  - Markedly diminished interest in and reduced ability to experience pleasure in almost all activities
  - Appetite increase or decrease resulting in significant weight loss or gain
  - Sleep disturbances (problems falling asleep, staying asleep, or sleeping too much)
  - Feeling or being restless or very slowed down
  - Fatigue, low energy
  - Feelings of worthlessness, guilt
  - Inability to concentrate, make decisions
  - Recurrent thoughts of death or suicide[6]
- If you are feeling any of these symptoms, PLEASE **contact your pastor or a Christian, Spirit-filled counselor.**
  - People who are trained in dealing with depression from a Biblical standpoint can give you guidance, help you change the aspects of your life that led to your depression, and pray with you for God's healing.

DEPRESSION OFTEN RUNS in families and many members of these families suffer from addiction.

- Some people become addicted in their attempts to abbreviate the problems of depression, including the emotional pain.
- All addictive substances, from sugar to narcotics, provide a temporary, *harmful* relief from depression.
  - Addictive substances act on the central nervous system— stimulating you (caffeine, amphetamines), depressing you

(sleeping pills, tranquilizers), or altering your perception (narcotics, marijuana).

■ Addiction is psychologically harmful because dependency creates more negative emotions (guilt, worthlessness, feeling out of control), and keeps you in a vicious, destructive cycle.

- Addictive people can become addicted to non-chemical activities such as work, exercise, gambling, or sex because the actions alleviate the symptoms of depression.
- Depression must be adequately treated before the addiction can be treated.[7]

YOU MAY ALLEVIATE the symptoms of depression or even eliminate the disorder by improving your diet and/or taking supplements of essential nutrients that are missing in the majority of chronically depressed patients. Depression is one of the early signs of nutritional depletion.

- Crash diets or starvation cause a deficiency of calories and nutrients.
- When you allow your blood sugar to fall too low (by not eating breakfast, skipping meals, etc.), you may become depressed.
- If you are allergic to certain foods and you continue to eat them, you can become depressed.[8]

IF YOU ARE chronically depressed, seek the advice of a trained, Christian, Spirit-filled counselor as well as following some of the suggestions listed below.

- Eat a well-balanced diet (see GUIDELINES TO HEALTHY EATING). When your body receives all the nutrients it needs to function properly, you will halt the majority of depression's symptoms.[9]

  ■ A diet deficient in vitamin B1 can depress your emotions and make you irritable, blue, or depressed.

    * Vitamin B1 (thiamin) is often called the morale vitamin because studies have shown it to elevate the moods

of many depressed people.[10]

- Triptophane (a chemical that converts into seratonin, a neural transmitter which calms the brain) prevents and combats depression.[11]
- Vitamin B6 is needed for your body to use triptophane properly.
  - Women who take birth control pills occasionally fall into deep depressions because the oral contraceptive creates a deficiency of vitamin B6.[12]
- A deficiency of vitamin B12 (which also causes a severe form of anemia) underlies most severe depression.[13]
- Vitamin C can ward off depression.[14]
- A shortage of iron will drain your energy and make you depressed.[15]
- A McGill University study found levels of folic acid far below normal in depressed patients.[16]
- Depression can be the first symptom of failure of the thyroid gland (an organ that regulates metabolism).
  - When your thyroid is starved of iodine (a nutrient the gland requires to function), it will rob you of energy and depress your emotions.
    - * If you are a first-generation hypothyroid (which means you are the first person in your family to have a low-functioning thyroid), you can correct your problem with an iodine-rich kelp tablet daily.
    - * If you are a second-generation hypothyroid (which means one of your parents or grandparents have a low-functioning thyroid), you can overcome the symptoms of the condition, including depression, by taking thyroid medicine prescribed by your physician.[17]
- Exercise helps battle depression.
- Live in a bright, cheerful, and sunlit place.
  - If you can't control the amount of sunlight in your home or you can't afford to replace your dark furnishings with

lighter colors, do other things that promote a "bright" lifestyle, such as taking walks in safe parks, spending a limited amount of time in the sun (always protecting your skin with sunblock, hats, or clothing), and surrounding yourself with positive people.

- Keep busy to alleviate symptoms of depression.
  - Activities can be individual and personal, such as reading, sewing, gardening, and redecorating; or creative and expressive, such as watercolors, oil painting, photography, and music.
- Love yourself.
  - Jesus said you should love your neighbors in the same way you love yourself (Matthew 19:19).[18]
- Keep in touch with your feelings.
  - People who are in control of their environment are less inclined to use and abuse chemicals such as alcohol and drugs.
- Think healthy.
- Celebrate life with renewed respect for your body, soul, and spirit.
  - Be aware of and careful with your body and what you put in it.[19]

WHEN GOD CREATED this world and all that resides in it, He gave everything a time to grow, to blossom, to tire, and to rest. He didn't create you any differently (Ecclesiastes 3:1-4).

- Like animals and plants, your body goes through changes of growth, reproduction, decay, and death.
  - Similar to what happens to your body, when your emotions are nurtured and given a healthy environment in which to grow, you will want to share your positive feelings with other people.
    * This sharing will give people a healthy, safe environment in which they can experience a positive emotional development.

* In other words, your positive emotions have reproduced.

■ If any of your emotions are not nurtured or developed, you will become sad and fearful, which may lead to seclusion or death.

• God will always nurture your emotions when you seek Him out; He will move on other people's hearts when you pray so you can receive help; and He will help you meet your heart's needs (Psalms 138:3).

■ You are a child of God, bought with a remarkable sacrifice, and offered an inheritance of hope, peace, joy, love, and eternal life (John 1:12).

■ God has a special purpose for your life (I Corinthians 2:9; 7:24).

■ God is always with you (Matthew 28:20).

■ God never forgets you (Romans 11:2).

■ You are **loved** (John 15:9).

■ Through Jesus, you are **victorious** (Romans 8:37)!

Section Six

CHANGE OF LIFE? MAKE IT A CHANGE FOR THE BETTER!

The passing to another stage of life happens to *every* woman. Shame, fear, misfortune, and the stigma of aging in a youth-obsessed society are some of the reasons women have kept silent about a passage that could not be more universal among females.

Menopause in previous eras was known as the "last taboo." Even in today's society, some women will tell a stranger about their innermost secrets, yet they shrink from mentioning the fear they might be menopausal.[1]

This is a *new day* and answers are more than readily available for today's woman as she approaches one of the most important periods of her life.

THE LAST TABOO

MENOPAUSE IS NOT a disease. It is the "final cessation of menstruation."[2]

- In the Greek, *meno* means "month," and *pausis* is translated "ending."[3]
    - Another name for menopause is the "Change of Life."
- It is a gradual start-stop series of pauses in the ovarian function that is part of the aging process.
- A more comprehensive term is "climacteric" (a period of decrease of reproductive capacity in men and women, culminating in women in the menopause).
- It's a life transition that carries with it a different internal hormonal makeup which can be detrimental to a woman's

body.

- There is a gradual loss of estrogen and other hormones until the ovaries stop putting out very much estrogen at all.
  - It is not uncommon for a woman to begin seeing symptoms in her early forties as a sign of gradual estrogen withdrawal.

WOMEN ARE BORN with all the eggs they'll ever have (about 700,000).

- Each month after puberty, one ovary offers up a selection of 20 to 1,000 mature eggs.
- Usually only one egg is released into the fallopian tube each month to meet any sperm in the vicinity.
  - Ovulation doesn't always take place as women get close to the bottom of their "egg basket."
- The quality of egg follicles released that month may be substandard, or there may not be sufficient estrogen manufactured by the ovaries.
- When the supply of viable eggs is gone, menstruation stops completely and the fertile period of a woman's life ends.[4]

AGE AND THE CHANGE OF LIFE

THE BIOLOGICAL TRANSITION of menopause is no longer an age-tied marker event.

- The median age for menopause is 50 to 58.
- There are no clear age cues as to when the menopausal transition begins or ends.
- A woman may never be quite sure when or if she has finished menopause.
  - This is particularly true for women who immediately begin hormone therapy at the first signs of menopause and continue having periods as if they were still reproductive.[5]

STATISTICS REVEAL THAT today's American women who are

visiting menopause clinics are four to five years younger than their predecessors were when they entered menopause a decade ago.

- Researchers now admit they've underestimated the number of younger women (some as early as their late thirties), who experience all the symptoms of menopause even though they still have monthly menstruation.[6]

MENOPAUSE CAN BE triggered by acute or prolonged stress, the removal of the ovaries, or the aging process.[7]

- It used to be that a reliable guide to when a woman might expect menopause was when her mother experienced it.
- The mothers of today's ground-breaking women did not experience the level of work-place stress and environmental toxins women live in today.
- Acute, prolonged, or severe stress can reduce the ovarian function and precipitate a temporary menopause at any time from the late thirties on.[8]

CHEMOTHERAPY CAN ALSO cause an immature menopause.

- Some women resume cycling naturally once the chemotherapy ends.[9]

THIRTY-SEVEN WOMEN out of 100 have hysterectomies (the removal of the uterus and cervix).

- The majority are between the ages of 25 and 44.
- A hysterectomy alone rarely produces menopause.
  - The removal of the ovaries (oophorectomy) brings on menopause immediately, no matter how young the woman is.

THE SUBTLE TRANSITION

NOTHING PREPARES MOST women for this mysterious and momentous transition.[10]

- Approximately 10 to 15 percent of women have no problems with menopause.
- Approximately 10 to 15 percent of menopausal women are

rendered temporarily dysfunctional.

- Seventy percent of women wrestle to some degree with difficulties that come and go over a period of years as they deal with changes in their reproductive state.[11]
- The next decade will see an explosion in the menopausal population in the U.S. because the number of women between the ages of 45 and 54 will increase by half.[12]

CULTURAL ATTITUDES

ATTITUDES AND REACTIONS to menopause vary significantly depending on how women are valued in a particular subculture.

- The "Change of Life" is experienced differently depending on one's cultural assumptions about aging, femininity, and the societal role of the older woman.
- 65 percent of Japanese women consider menopause as uneventful.
  - The Japanese language doesn't have a word for hot flashes.
  - In China, age is venerated and menopausal symptoms are rarely reported.
- In America, youth and desirability go hand-in-hand, and the role for the older woman is uncertain.
- Although menopause in the U.S. is defined in almost hormonal terms, cultural attitudes cast the signs and symptoms in a negative light.[13]

MENOPAUSE DIFFERS WITH EACH INDIVIDUAL

MENOPAUSE IN AMERICA differs with each woman.

- The older a woman becomes, the more *unlike* she is from others.

- In addition to the changes in her brain and sexual characteristics over the years, her endocrine system and metabolism are different; her blood vessels and bones become more dissimilar, depending on her lifetime eating and exercise habits.
- It is not surprising that there is not one menopause; rather there are hundreds of variations.[14]

SOME WOMEN ARE naturally nervous when approaching menopause about letting go of aspects of their femininity.

- They become more acutely aware of health, appearance, economic security, and mortality.[15]

SECOND ADULTHOOD

THE "CHANGE OF Life" is one of the three great "blood mysteries" that mark a woman's inner life, the earlier ones being menarche (the beginning of menstruation), and pregnancy.[16]

- Menopause is no longer a marker that means "This way to the end."
- Age 50 is the apex of the female life cycle.
- Menopause is more properly seen today as the gateway to a second adulthood (a series of stages never before part of the predictable life cycle for other than the very long-lived).

THERE ARE THREE stages of the second adulthood.

- *Perimenopause* (the start of the ovarian transition between regular periods and no periods at all); *menopause* (completion of the ovarian transition); and *coalescence* (the exact opposite of adolescence in which women can tap into the new vitality called postmenopausal zest).[17]
- The number of women in perimenopause, menopause, or coalescence in the U.S. totals about 43 million.[18]

PERIMENOPAUSE'S FIRST SIGN is very often gushing (a sudden heavy flow of blood that may be dark or clotted and that may seep through a woman's normal protection).

- Almost every woman bleeds erratically during perimenopause.

PERIMENOPAUSE BEGINS WHEN a woman stops ovulating every month.

- The months when ovulation doesn't occur, a woman's body doesn't produce progesterone (the hormone ordinarily responsible for flushing the lining of the uterus).
    - The endometrial lining becomes thicker and may not be entirely flushed until the next cycle, when the body releases the previous month's buildup.
- One month a woman may have a heavy period, and the next month she may not have a period at all.
- Other symptoms of perimenopause may be the development of cysts in her breast, or functional ovarian cysts.
- Two months or a year later she may be back to "normal."
    - The reason for all the fluctuation is because the hormone levels are surging and falling in frantic response to desperate signals from the brain to the pituitary.
    - The menstrual cycle not only becomes erratic but is uncoupled from the change in temperature and sleep cycles; and can affect the woman's appetite, sexual interest, and overall sense of well-being.
    - The body's whole balance is thrown off.
    - While this can be very unsettling, it is a temporary phenomenon.

A WOMAN SHOULD not allow herself to be railroaded into a hysterectomy or onto hormones.

- Her body will be out of sync with its own chemistry for two to three years.[19]

THE RAGING HORMONES of adolescence suddenly become the unraging hormones of menopause.

- Most women after menopause, if they're reasonably healthy and happy, do not experience a decrease in their sex drive (30 percent do).[20]

- The lessening of sexual desire is related to vaginal dryness, which suggests both hormonal and psychological factors.
- The lack of interest in sex may also be due to a decrease in testosterone (the male sex hormone that women's bodies produce in very small quantities).
  - Testosterone levels decrease in some women beyond the fourth or fifth year of menopause.

TESTOSTERONE IS COMMONLY reported as the hormone primarily responsible for sexual motivation in women, just as it is in men.

- In approximately 50 percent of women, the ovaries stop producing testosterone around the time of menopause.
- In another 50 percent they go on functioning, and in some women the ovaries go on overtime, producing more testosterone than during their reproductive life.
  - These are the women who notice some hair appearing on their upper lips or chins.[21]

MENOPAUSE IS THE second stage of second adulthood.

- It is one of the most difficult phases of a woman's life.
- It is characterized by backaches, breathing difficulties, depression, dizziness, excessive menstrual flow, fatigue, headaches, hot flashes and inordinate sweating, nervousness and heart palpitations, and dry vaginal tissues.[22]
  - One-half of all women who have hot flashes will begin feeling them while they are still menstruating (some as early as age 40).
  - Studies show most women have hot flashes for two years.
  - One-fourth of all women experience hot flashes for five years; ten percent will experience hot flashes for the rest of their lives.[23]

THE HIDDEN THIEVES of menopause include heart disease, osteoporosis (a loss of bone density), cognitive changes (such as memory loss), and cancer.

- This knowledge must be factored in *before* a woman can

make an intelligent decision about how to best manage her own menopause.

HEART DISEASE IS the number one menopause thief and killer of women over 50.

- A woman's chances of dying from heart disease are more than double that of dying from cancer of any kind.
- Cardiovascular disease quietly kills one in two women over the age of 50.

THE RATE OF heart disease rises sharply for women 50 years and older.

- Women lag behind men in heart disease by about five to seven years.
- By the age of 67, women are just as likely to have heart attacks as men the same age, but women are more likely to die from them.

HIGH-DENSITY LIPOPROTEIN (HDL—good cholesterol level) is the most significant predictor of heart disease.

- Bad cholesterol levels (LDL) normally increase in women for some ten to fifteen years following the cessation of periods.
- Dangerous changes in cholesterol count or blood pressure do not announce themselves with obvious symptoms.
  - Estrogen replacement therapy decreases LDL (low-density lipoprotein) cholesterol levels and raises the HDL cholesterol levels, each by about 15 percent.

ESTROGEN HAS A direct effect on the wall of the blood vessels.

- An increase in cholesterol is the first change that occurs in the formation of the plaque in arteries.
- Estrogen appears to block that effect, resulting in open vessels and good blood flow.
- Estrogen reduces the risk of heart disease.[24]

OSTEOPOROSIS IS THE second major thief of menopause.

- A woman is never too *young* to start protecting her bones.
- Women begin losing bone density after the age of 35.

- The normal rate of loss is about one percent a year.
- The loss of bone density accelerates to about 1-1/2 percent each year once a woman turns 50.
- It then levels off again at one percent a year.

A WOMAN'S GENETIC background and her bone strength determine her risk of bone density loss during this transition.

- About one-third of American women of all ages are calcium-deficient.
- Bones with an excess of pores lead to an increased risk of fractures.
  - Porous bones are a major public health problem for one-third to one-half of all postmenopausal women.
- Nearly half of all women over age 75 will be affected by osteoporosis.

WOMEN DIE FROM the consequences of osteoporosis.

- It often leaves older women frail, susceptible to falls and broken bones, as well as to the little tortures of hairline fractures in the bones they use for walking and bending.

CALCIUM SUPPLEMENTS ALONE cannot undo the damage done by the loss of estrogen during this period of accelerated loss.

- Exercise by itself is also ineffective in preventing osteoporosis.
- An exercise program plus calcium supplements slow or stop bone density loss.
- The best results are obtained when estrogen is combined with exercise.
  - Bone mass is increased and other symptoms such as hot flashes and sleeplessness diminish.

VITAMIN K INHIBITS the loss of calcium in postmenopausal women.

- Dark green leafy vegetables like broccoli and Brussels sprouts are sources of vitamin K.
- Exercise such as brisk walking or walking on a treadmill at a tilt provides both weight bearing and aerobic benefits.[25]

MEMORY LOSS CAUSED by estrogen deprivation is another thief of menopause.

- Estrogen helps to increase the blood flow to the brain.
- The absence of estrogen has a powerful effect on synapses at certain sites in the brain.
- Estrogen has an effect on mental functioning (not on IQ but in terms of performance).[26]

BREAST CANCER PHOBIA has overtaken almost all other health issues surrounding menopause for many American women.[27]

- One in nine women are diagnosed with breast cancer.
- The risk of getting breast cancer rises steadily with age in all women, including those who are not secreting estrogen or taking it in replacement hormones.[28]

MENOPAUSE AND MEDICINE

SOME WOMEN RESIST medicalizing a natural event such as menopause. Others have little choice.

- Many experts are now openly promoting estrogen replacement therapy.
- Some top researchers are even reversing themselves on the conventional prescription for combined hormone replacement therapy.[29]

THE STANDARDIZED PRESCRIPTION for menopause is 0.625 mg of Premarin (estrogen made from pregnant mares' urine), and 10 mg tablets of Provera (the progestin that stimulates the sloughing or separation of the uterine lining).

- These are approximations of the two hormones that the body produces naturally in the reproductive years.

ESTROGEN REKINDLES SEXUAL desire.

- It stops the surges and dips in the energy level and chases away depression.[30]
- If a woman does not take estrogen, her bones will become brittle, her risk of heart disease increases, her vagina will

become atrophied (less moist), and her skin will become dry and thin.

PROGESTIN INDUCES PHYSICAL and emotional symptoms and causes the body to be at war within itself.[31]

- Doctors report that progestin blocks some of the estrogen-receptor sites—so the woman experiences a literal war between the two hormones.
- Progestin counters some of the cardio-protective effects that are a major benefit of estrogen.
- Unlike estrogen, progestin offers no added protection against bone loss.

PROGESTIN PROTECTS THE uterus.[32]

- Estrogen used alone has been clearly linked with an increased incidence of uterine cancer.
- Abnormal bleeding patterns may forewarn of precancerous changes in the lining of the uterus.
- These early signs DON'T ALWAYS occur.

THESE POWERFUL HORMONES cross the blood-brain bridge.

- Sensors in the brain that control emotions pick up a signal when there is an erratic production of either estrogen or progesterone.
- In a person whose nervous system is finely tuned, these sensors overreact, triggering brain-chemistry changes and emotional upheaval.

THERE ARE AT least a dozen different regimens recommended by doctors for combining estrogen and progestin.

- No two women respond the same way.
- Estrogen affects the heart, mind, bones, behavior, and sexual function and desire.
- Some studies indicate that women live longer if they are on estrogen.[33]
    - A recent study revealed the longer a woman used estrogen replacement therapy, the lower her early mortality risk.

QUESTIONS WOMEN SHOULD ASK THEMSELVES BEFORE MENOPAUSE

WOMEN SHOULD ANSWER the following questions to assist their doctors in taking care of them:

- Is there any evidence of osteoporosis in my family?
- Did my mother or a sister have breast cancer? At what age? Was it estrogen-sensitive?
- Is there a family history of heart disease?
- Is there a family history of cancer of the uterus?
- How long have I been perimenopausal? (The longer it takes a woman to move from irregular cycles to no cycles, the more likely she is to have physical and emotional symptoms.)
- On a scale of one to ten, what concerns me most about menopause?
  - If a woman has had a pre-cancerous condition in her cervix, she should not worry; cervical cancer is not hormone-dependent. There is no evidence that estrogen increases the risk of ovarian cancer.[34]

HORMONE REPLACEMENT THERAPY

THE DISADVANTAGES OF hormone replacement therapy include:

1) A possible increased risk of cancer of the uterus
2) Unknown associations with breast cancer
3) Continued menstruation
4) Breast swelling or pain
5) Premenstrual-like syndrome
6) The expense of doctor's visits and tests for screening

THE ADVANTAGES OF hormone replacement therapy include:

1) It prevents osteoporosis.
2) It decreases the risk of heart attacks.

3) It eliminates hot flashes.

4) It decreases insomnia.

5) It improves the energy level.

6) It improves a woman's mood and sense of well-being.

7) It restores sexual interest.

BEWARE OF OLD wives' tales such as, "Once a woman starts on hormones she will have to stay on them forever."

- Larger doses of hormones may be required to control a woman's symptoms when she *first* begins menopause.
- As she gets older, the medication can be reduced because her body will be more tolerant of the decreased dosage.
- Women should avoid going off hormones "cold turkey."
    - The more abrupt the drop in these hormones, the more severe the symptoms.
    - Taper off![35]

NATURAL METHODS OF TREATMENT

WHILE FEMALE HORMONES are often used to relieve symptoms—with the risk of contributing to cancer—certain safe nutrients have been shown to be helpful.

- Primrose oil can be used to relieve hot flashes because it contains gamma-linolenic acid, which helps regulate hormonal activity.
- Vitamin E is commonly used to reduce hot flashes.
    - Vitamin E is also helpful for the menopausal complaint of atrophied (dry) vaginal tissues.
    - The symptoms of an atrophied vagina include a lack of lubrication, itching, and pain during sexual intercourse.
- One of the best natural defenses against osteoporosis is to keep the acidity of the blood in proper balance.
    - The body balances itself naturally by removing calcium

from the bones to defend the pH balance in the blood.

- Blood acidity is caused, first and foremost, by chronic stress.
  - Women 45 years and older who are faced with high stress professional or personal demands should commit themselves to some restorative relaxation measures.
  - Smoking, alcohol, and coffee also increase the acid levels in the blood.
  - Carbonated sodas and beef, both of which have a high phosphorus content, are particularly dangerous for postmenopausal women.
  - A suggested diet should emphasize vegetables, complex carbohydrates, fiber, fish, and vegetable proteins such as tofu.

AN EXPERIMENTAL STUDY revealed the greater effectiveness of the citrus-derived bioflavonoids hesperiden and hesperiden methyl chalcone in relieving certain symptoms of menopause (mainly gushing) than sub-therapeutic dosages of estrogen and similar treatments.

- Emotional storms in menopause (including nervousness and depression) are often quieted with vitamin B-complex (plus brewer's yeast, liver, other organ meats, wheat germ and whole grains), bioflavonoids, lecithin, calcium, and vitamin E.

SOME DOCTORS BELIEVE menopausal problems can often be handled without using female hormones, which can over-stimulate responsive tissues such as the breast and uterus, contributing to cancer.

THE FOLLOWING ARE some supplements and foods with the highest ratings of vitamin E in International Units per less than four-ounce portions:

- Wheat germ, 160; safflower nuts, 35; sunflower seeds, 31; whole wheat, 30; sesame oil, 26; walnuts, 22; corn oil and hazelnuts, 21; soy oil and peanut oil, 16; almonds, 15; olive oil, 14; cabbage, 7.8; brazil nuts and peanuts, 6.5; cod liver oil, 5.4; cashews, 5.1; soy lecthin, 4.8; spinach, 2.9; asparagus, 2.5; broccoli, 2.0; butter, 1.9; parsley, 1.8; and oats, barley and corn, 1.7

THE BEST SUPPLEMENTS and food sources of calcium are: bone meal, 40,000; dolomite, 21,000; sesame seeds, 1,200; kelp, 1.100; cheeses, 700; brewer's yeast, 420; sardines and carob, 350; molasses, 290; caviar, 280; soybeans and almonds, 230; torula yeast, 220; parsley, 200; brazil nuts, 190; watercress, salmon, and chickpeas, 150; egg yolk, beans, pistachios, lentils and kale, 130; sunflower seeds and milk, 120; buckwheat, 110; maple syrup, cream, and chard, 100; walnuts, 99; spinach, 93; endive, 81; and pecans, 73.[36]

COALESCENCE

COALESCENCE MARKS THE end of the ovarian transition.
- Women enter a new state of equilibrium.
- Their energy, moods, and overall sense of physical and mental well-being should be restored, but with a difference.

COALESCENCE MEANS "TO come together," or "to unite."
- This is a time when all the wisdom a woman has gathered from 50 years of experience in living comes together.
- She has a second chance in postmenopause, unencumbered by the day-to-day caregiving.
- She is free to focus on the things she loves most and to redirect her creativity.
- She can rediscover who she really is and plot a new direction for her life.[37]

MENOPAUSE AND YOUR ATTITUDE

WOMEN WHO MAINTAIN a right attitude through the various changes of their lives, and hold onto the Word of God, will come through menopause very well.
- Sarah experienced menopause (Genesis 18:11).
- Perhaps some of the problems she had with Hagar were due

to the changes her body was experiencing in menopause. EVERY WOMAN CAN overcome menopause if she takes the Word of God into her "change" with her.

- The Word is changeless and can change a person's attitude.
- God's Word can even change the hormone level.
- The way a woman attacks symptoms of menopause with the Bible is going to determine her outcome.

A WOMAN'S ATTITUDE affects her body (see WINNING OVER THE WEIGHTS OF LIFE and SHEDDING THE HABITS THAT WEIGH YOU DOWN).

- A woman's attitude determines how she responds to the changes taking place in her body.
- Spend a lot of time in the Word and in prayer.
- What happens in the mind and emotions, through the effect of God's Word and the power of His Holy Spirit, will determine the success of a woman's menopause.

SOME WOMEN (LIKE Sarah) carry the weight of the change in a terrible way and it will weigh them down.

- Cast the weight of menopause on the Lord (I Peter 5:7).
- The female physical body may change, but God's Word does not change (Malachi 3:6).

Section Seven
RAISING HEALTHY KIDS IN A JUNK-FOOD WORLD

Every phase of your life brings changes. The nine months you were in the womb was a time of **major** change. You grew from a *single cell* to a human being with arteries, veins, nerves, organs, arms, legs, fingers, and toes. That is remarkable! As an adult, you have about 700 trillion cells in your body, all regulated by enzymes, hormones, and various chemicals that fulfill specific roles to keep you alive.

Through messages sent along your nervous system, your brain controls the rate of your development; stores your memories; determines your speech patterns; regulates your moods; establishes your intelligence; and processes every bit of information you receive through touch, taste, smell, hearing, and sight.

With all of these processes going on at the same time, the miracle of life isn't so much that you were born, but that your body can tolerate daily abuses—whether you smoke, drink alcohol, overeat, live in a polluted area, experience a high level of stress, take drugs or medications, or remain idle.

I want to walk through the various stages of a body's growth and give you some tips on what kinds of foods and activities will help you combat some of the problems, illnesses, or diseases that can come upon you during childhood, adolescence, and young adulthood. Read all the sections because some of the complaints people have in their middle and senior years could have been prevented in their childhood or teen years. And remember, through it all, God is one of grace and mercy. Search His Word, communicate with Him through prayer, and stay active doing the things God has called you to do.

CHILD

Babies grow rapidly. They enter the world at around 7 pounds and reach 21 to 35 pounds by the time they are 2 years old. That's three to five times their original size in two years! Children vary in size, but always check with your pediatrician about whether your child is too heavy or too little for his age. It's hard to determine on your own if your child is within healthy limits; however, most children weigh between 60 and 125 pounds by their twelfth year.

MAKE SURE YOUR baby receives all the nutrients she needs.

- Many nursing mothers believe that despite their own poor health and undernourishment, their breast milk will sustain their infant in good health.
  - Good nutrition will produce good mother's milk, and poor nutrition will produce poor mother's milk. [1]
  - When breastfeeding, a mother needs to daily take in (through supplements and/or food) 25,000 IU of vitamin A; a vitamin B-complex capsule; 1,000 mg vitamin C; 25 to 50 IU of vitamin E; Vitamin K (from three or four Brussels sprouts, a bowl of oatmeal, or several ounces of spinach, or broccoli); 18 to 20 mg iron (from three or four ounces of pumpkin seeds and a bowl of wheat germ cereal); 1,200 mg calcium; 400 IU of vitamin D (from a tablespoon of cod liver oil or several ounces of sardines or salmon); and 600 to 700 mg of magnesium (from four ounces of sunflower seeds and a bowl of wheat germ cereal). [2]
    - * During the nursing stage, calcium requirements are higher than at any other time of life because the mother must supply her own needs and those of the baby. Taking in less than 1,200 mg can cause osteoporosis after menopause. [3]
  - A nursing mother's protein intake should be 10 percent more than during pregnancy. An extra slice of whole grain

bread and a few ounces of almonds, cashews, or sunflower seeds will provide the added protein.[4]

- Mother's milk has numerous advantages over cow and soy milk.
  - It contains colostrum (which is the first milk from the mother's breast and gives the baby the mother's immunity from the flu, polio, staph infections, and other viruses).
  - It has more zinc (important for a strong immune system, rapid healing, and proper sexual development).
  - It is easier for the baby to digest.
  - It is less likely to cause celiac disease (a disorder characterized by a defect in digestion, preventing absorption of fat and calcium).[5]
- Healthy breast-fed infants take in fewer calories and grow at a different rate than healthy bottle-fed babies.[6]

WOMEN CAN PASS along the effects of drugs, medicines, and other substances in their breast milk, which can jeopardize the baby's health.

- Even when a drug isn't toxic, it could cause allergies in the baby or drastic changes in friendly, intestinal tract bacteria.[7]
  - Alcohol should be eliminated.
  - Amphetamines could disturb the baby's sleep and leave her irritable.
  - Antibiotics upset the balance of friendly and unfriendly bacteria in the large intestine.
  - Antihistamines, decongestants, and medicines for bronchitis or asthma may bring on crying, irritability or sleeplessness in the baby.
  - Aspirin could interfere with the baby's ability to clot blood.
  - Barbituates and certain sleeping pills can cause the baby to sleep too deeply or too long.
  - Caffeine can make the baby irritable and unable to sleep.[8]

PREPARED FORMULA COMES in milk- and soy-based varieties, because some babies are allergic to cow's milk.

- Prepare powdered and concentrated formulas according to the container's or your doctor's directions.
  - Diluted (weak) formula will deprive your baby of the nourishment she needs.[9]
- To avoid infection, always use sterilized bottles and nipples when preparing the formula.
  - A baby who fusses soon after starting a bottle may be frustrated because the nipple hole is too small or clogged.
    * Simply use a different nipple.
  - Bottle-fed babies are more likely to have gastroenteritis than breast-fed babies, partly because the bottles and nipples may not be properly sterilized.
    * Gastroenteritis is an illness that causes the stomach and small intestine to become inflamed. The baby will have loose, green, watery bowel movements (diarrhea) and will sometimes vomit.
    * The disorder may be nothing more than a mild stomach upset, or it may be a severe attack that leads to dehydration.
      □ In mild cases, the baby remains happy and eats well. In more severe attacks, the baby is miserable and irritable, eats poorly, has a slight fever, and may vomit. A baby who has as many as 10 bowel movements in a day may become dehydrated.
        ★ Signs of dehydration are a dry mouth, sunken eyes and fontanel (the baby's soft spot), lethargy, irritability, and in some cases vomiting back all fluids. In severe dehydration (a DANGEROUS condition), the baby's skin will not immediately return to its original position when you gently pinch it between your thumb and finger. In addition, the baby refuses to eat and may have

a fever or a below-normal temperature. If dehydration reaches an advanced stage, it can cause brain damage or even death.[10]

SOME BABIES MAY cry after they eat.

- A baby will nearly always swallow some air (whether she is breast or bottle fed). Pat the baby's back gently but firmly until she burps up the air.
- Cuddle the baby. If she has had enough nourishment, she will go to sleep.[11]
- If your baby seems to get enough breast milk but still seems to be hungry and irritable, try this experiment: give her a bottle after she has nursed both breasts.
    - If she drinks three to four ounces, you probably don't have enough milk. Contact your doctor to see if you have a declining milk supply or other problem.
        - * If your milk supply is declining, sometimes it can be rejuvenated by more frequent feedings.
            - ☐ Other causes of lowered milk production are the Pill, which is harmful to milk and infant; heavy smoking of cigarettes and marijuana; an elevated fever; low thyroid function; fatigue; or pregnancy.[12]
            - ☐ Mothers of premature infants (8 to 12 weeks early) should pump both breasts empty at least six times a day.[13]
- If the baby continues to cry, or cries a lot between feedings, she may not be getting enough to eat.
    - A sign of inadequate feeding is that the baby has small, firm, dark green bowel movements.
    - Try to give the baby more to eat. Don't worry about overfeeding; the baby knows when to stop.
    - Some babies cry because they are thirsty, especially in hot weather. Try giving your baby some water in a bottle.[14]
- During the first few weeks of life, some babies start to eat

actively, then drop off to sleep. When this happens, wake the baby and stimulate her to start eating again.

- ■ The phase passes in a healthy baby, but if it continues, she may have an infection, and you should see your doctor.
- • If your baby begins to eat slowly for four or five days after having eaten normally, talk to your pediatrician.[15]

MOST BABIES SPIT up a little milk, particularly when they burp. This is especially true of bottle-fed babies, because the bottles may have the wrong-sized nipples, which causes the baby to swallow a lot of air.

- • Very active babies regurgitate often.
  - ■ Spitting up usually stops when the baby is given solid foods at four to six months.
- • It usually stops completely around nine months old.
- • Vomiting, rather than spitting up, may be due to a disorder.
  - ■ Check with your doctor, especially if the vomit shoots some distance.[16]

YOUR BABY WILL probably be ready for solid foods when she is four to six months old.

- • Talk to your pediatrician about the types and kinds of foods your baby can eat and how to handle situations in which she is allergic or unable to tolerate certain foods.
- • Once your baby has been introduced to a variety of foods, such as eggs, soft fruit and vegetables, and milk puddings, the amount of milk you give should be reduced; otherwise she may become overweight.
- • Start your baby off with good eating habits!
  - ■ Try to limit the amount of refined sugar and flour products you feed her—for snacks try fruit or whole grain breads or muffins.
  - ■ Don't use food to pacify your child when she is emotionally upset.[17]

WHEN YOUR CHILD is ready for "adult" foods, make sure he is introduced to a full spectrum of vegetables, fruit, meats, grains, and nuts, prepared in a variety of ways.

- If your child is a picky eater, don't cater to his demands, especially when he wants only one type of food all the time or will eat only sugary, salty, junk foods.
  - Dinnertime should always be peaceful, not only for the family's digestion and health, but also because food will become an issue with your child, not a source of nourishment.
- Make your child's food more inviting.
  - One idea for breakfast is to arrange pancakes or waffles on the plate to resemble a mouse, with smaller rounds as the ears and the larger round as the face. Decorate with fresh (not sugared) fruit, with blueberries as eyes, pineapple triangles as a bowtie, strawberries as the mouth, etc.
- Your child will be more likely to eat a meal in which he had a hand in preparing.
  - Young children can put already-chopped vegetables into a soup or salad.
  - Teach older children to chop vegetables (under your supervision, this process will give them the extra ability to handle sharp objects correctly) and create salads.
  - Let your children help you plan healthful meals, make grocery lists, etc.
  - To make even the most vegetable-phobic child eager to eat carrots or broccoli, let them grow their own vegetables. It is more likely that a child will eat what he has helped grow and prepare.

JUVENILE ONSET DIABETES (called Type I Diabetes) occurs in children when the pancreas produces very little or no insulin.

- It is a myth that children who eat a lot of sugar will get diabetes.
  - The exact cause of diabetes is unknown, but it does not seem to be directly related to sugar. However, sugar is

not healthy for children and can lead to overweight, tooth decay, and hyperactivity.

- Type I Diabetes is treated with a combination of a controlled diet and daily injections of insulin to replace the missing hormone.
- If your child has Type I Diabetes, it is essential to teach her self-discipline so she can maintain her health.
- Ask your pediatrician if your child can engage in sports or any heavy exercise, since exercise burns up glucose and may bring on hypoglycemia.[18]

BEDWETTING IS A problem for many children. Sometimes the inability to control his bladder during the night will last a couple months after potty training or can reach into puberty in rare situations.

- Children who are unable to control their bladders may be deficient in the mineral magnesium.
  - Increase the amount of foods that are high in magnesium in your child's diet. A good amount is about 600 mg daily. Consult your doctor if you think your child should have supplements.
- Most children who wet the bed during the night have smaller bladders than other children.
  - Most bed-wetters overcome their problem by the time they are five—either through enlargement of the bladder or through receiving stronger physical signals to wake up and go to the bathroom.
- Your child may be allergic to the food she most often eats, causing the bladder to react by automatically emptying the urine to get rid of the offending food's residue.
- A useful folk remedy is to give your child a teaspoon of raw, unfiltered, unprocessed honey before bedtime.[19]

HYPERACTIVE CHILDREN OFTEN are restless, jittery, unable to concentrate or read; deliver below-average work; are unable to organize work or stay with projects; are impatient; touch everything and everybody around them; have a hair-trigger temper; are aggressive and disrupt the class and cause friction with classmates and teachers; are easy to bring to tears and depressed states; and have a hard time sleeping.

- This condition has been linked to the child having been undernourished during the first three years of life—including time in the womb.
  - Children may eat a lot and still not get enough nourishment because they don't eat enough healthful foods (see GUIDELINES FOR HEALTHY EATING).
- Drugs treat only the symptoms of hyperactivity and have potential side effects: chronic sleeplessness, irritability, loss of appetite and weight, nausea, tactile hallucinations, and tics (spasmodic and uncontrollable muscle contractions).
  - Long-time use of such drugs may result in brain damage, heart and artery disorders, Hodgkin's disease, and drug dependency.
- Don't feed your child junk foods.
  - A well-maintained diet will regulate your child's hyperactivity.
  - Cut out soft drinks, sugary baked goods, and bottled, canned, packaged, and processed foods (especially those with additives).
  - A diet high in refined carbohydrates triggers low blood sugar—a condition called hypoglycemia—which can lead to hyperactivity.
- Hyperactivity can be caused by your child's allergies to common foods (usually the foods he eats most often).
- Vitamin B6 activates enzymes which convert tryptophan (an amino acid) into serotonin. Blood tests of hyperactive people showed they have below-normal levels of serotonin, and when given vitamin B6 their serotonin levels rose and their hyperactivity ceased.
  - Give your child plenty of foods high in vitamin B6: brewer's

yeast, brown rice, whole wheat, soybeans, rye, lentils, sunflower seeds, hazelnuts, alfalfa, salmon, wheat germ, tuna, bran, walnuts, peas, liver, avocados, beans, cashews, peanuts, oats, beef, chicken, turkey, halibut, lamb, banana, blackstrap molasses, corn, and eggs.

- Many children have difficulty translating essential fatty acids (EFAs) in vegetable oils into prostaglandins (PGs), which are present in every human cell and vital to the function of every human organ.
  - Hyperactive boys outnumber hyperactive girls three to one, perhaps because boys have a hard time converting EFAs into PGs.
  - Give your child a 500 mg capsule of Evening Primrose Oil in the morning and the evening. Also, rub the oil into your child's skin.
- Make sure your child gets a daily dose of vigorous, aerobic exercise.[20]

TEEN

Adolescence is the often difficult period of transition from childhood to adulthood. Many of the characteristic problems of adolescence stem from changes in the type and pattern of hormones present in the body.

Puberty begins with girls when they are 10 to 12 years old, and with boys it is around age 13 or 14. Physical maturity reaches a plateau at about the age of 17 or 18 in both sexes. During those intervening years, your teenager will undergo physical, mental, and emotional pressures that can make adolescence a particularly difficult time.

Make sure your teenager can come to you with any problem and that she has all the skills necessary for her to use God's Word to find her solutions. Give her guidance with her diet, and instill in her an understanding of her worth as a child of God. If her appearance is a major factor in her life, help her achieve her physical ideal if it is within realistic limits. Or help her redirect her goals if she might do herself harm through excessive dieting (See HEALTHY APPETITES FOR A LONG LIFE), steroid use, over exercise, harmful surgery, etc.

ACNE PLAGUES ALMOST every teenager to some extent. It is a source of embarrassment and can even hamper your teenager's social development.

- Almost the entire body is covered with hairs, most of them virtually invisible. Each hair grows from a follicle (a tiny pit in the skin) and within each follicle is a sebaceous gland that produces an oily substance called sebum that lubricates the skin. If there is an overproduction of oil and some of it becomes trapped in a follicle, bacteria can multiply in the blocked pit and cause it to become inflamed. The result is a pimple, which may be a red lump or may become a pus-filled whitehead.[21]
- Although it is a problem for some adults, acne begins at puberty and usually clears up in the late teens or early 20s.
  - The level of male hormones in the body rises when a boy or girl reaches puberty, and this stimulates the sebaceous glands to increase their production of sebum.[22]
- The first step to curing acne is keeping your skin clean. Wash it with an unscented soap two times a day.
  - Treat your skin carefully. Don't scrub or wash more than twice daily as it will cause your skin to dry and get flaky and may increase production of oils.
- Do not use creams or lotions unless they are prescribed or recommended by your doctor.
- A limited exposure to sunshine helps in many cases of acne, so spend as much time in the open air as possible.
- Girls should refrain from wearing foundation makeup.
- Don't squeeze the pustules because this can disfigure the face, leaving the skin scarred and pitted.
- Eat a diet high in zinc or take 50 to 100 mg supplements

of the mineral.
- Take a supplement of vitamin A.
- Be aware of food sensitivities and allergies, and cut out those foods which cause you problems.
- Eat a diet high in fresh vegetables and fruit, as well as some fish, poultry, meat, and eggs.[23]

ALCOHOL, CIGARETTES, AND drugs are dangerous for anyone; but teenagers are especially vulnerable to addiction. Adolescents tend to be attracted to rebellious activities, think they will live forever, are susceptible to peer pressure, and are searching for identities separate from their parents'.

- Drugs and other addictive substances are easily available to teenagers, making the temptations more widespread.
- Many teenagers try drugs, alcohol, and cigarettes to appear more adult, to cover up a feeling of social inadequacy, or to conform.
  - When a teenager tries one substance it may lead to trying another. This experimentation may lead to dependence, addiction, and death.
  - Statistics show that the majority of adults who are addicted to substances began using them in adolescence.[24]
- Alcohol use and abuse can cause a wide range of physical and mental problems, particularly in teenagers and young adults.
  - Alcohol can cause blackouts, brain damage, hallucinations, impaired vision, slurred speech, unsteadiness, staggering, coma, stupor, and strokes.
  - The majority of strokes and cerebral hemorrhages (fatal bleeding in the brain) that strike young people happen within 24 hours after a heavy drinking period.
  - Sometimes less than an ounce of alcohol causes arterioles (branches of arteries a little larger than capillaries) to spasm and to cut off oxygen to all parts of the body.
    * With a frequent and high intake of alcohol, arteriole

walls weaken and rupture under this extreme pressure.

   * Chronic alcoholics on a binge may experience a high rate of strokes, high blood pressure, and sudden death because of these weakened arterioles.[25]

- Educate your children about the effects of addictive substances, tell them the dangers of addiction, instill in them a recognition of their own self-worth, pay attention to signs of depression, and make sure they are receiving a diet filled with all the nutrients their bodies need.

   * Depression and addiction stem from a deficiency of many key nutrients[26] (see SHEDDING THE HABITS THAT WEIGH YOU DOWN).

YOUNG ADULT

By the time you've entered your 20s your bones have stopped growing and nearly every aspect of your personality has been established. Habits learned throughout your childhood and adolescence have become a lifestyle—your attitudes, diet, and exercise regime. You should know, however, that when you trust in God to help you make changes in your life, it is NEVER too late to break bad habits!

As a young adult you face more stress than you had growing up— you leave high school and/or college, move away from home, start and establish your career, create lifelong relationships, build your family, buy your first car and house, and start walking down the pathway to the rest of your life.

When faced with so many challenges, it's sometimes too easy to neglect your body, emotions, and spirituality. But it is important for you to make these three things your priority, because if any one of them fails, your future and that of your family may be devastated by illness, heartbreak, and despair. I encourage you to begin eating right, exercising, examining your feelings, setting aside time for prayer, and getting into God's Word. I can't think of a better foundation on which to build your life.

GUM AND TOOTH care takes lifelong dedication and requires much more than brushing and flossing teeth regularly and having a checkup and professional cleaning semi-annually. The biggest part of taking care of teeth and gums is proper nutrition.

- The widely accepted theory about tooth socket deterioration is that it starts with diseased gums. Harmful bacteria invade the gums and cause inflammation which then attacks the jawbone. However, studies have shown that bone loss through poor nutrition is actually what starts the deterioration process.
  - Only one percent of your body's calcium stores circulate in your blood and in the fluids between your cells, but that amount must be maintained at all cost. When you take in too little calcium through food or supplements, your body makes up for the shortage by drawing calcium out of your bones.
  - As calcium is withdrawn from your jawbone, your jaw will shrink (as this process continues it takes more and more calcium from your ribs, vertebrae, and arm and leg bones). As the jawbone and its tooth sockets shrink, bone pulls away from the teeth, causing them to loosen. This irritates and then inflames your gums and can cause bleeding.
- Vitamin C is a powerful agent for dental health because it helps build bones and heal gums.
  - Vitamin C helps form connective tissue, a weblike fiber that binds cells together. The connective tissue in gums firms up the flesh and keeps bacteria from penetrating into the tooth sockets and contributing to periodontal disease.
  - Vitamin C also helps correct soggy, sore, bleeding gums.
    * Longtime deficiencies of vitamin C make your gums watery and weak, leading to puffy gums.
- Vitamin A helps tear down old bone tissue, dissolve and

134

dispose of dead bone wastes, and form new bone tissues.
- ■ Abnormal bone formations may occur if you are deficient of vitamin A.
- You should take 1,200 mg a day of calcium; 400 IU of vitamin D; 10,000 IU of vitamin A; 600 mg of magnesium; 30 mg of zinc; and 1,500 mg of vitamin C.
  - ■ This regime will reduce gum inflammation and may eliminate the problem. Loose teeth will tighten up and may return to normal as the size of the jawbone increases and fills in some bone which had parted from the tooth roots.[27]

ANEMIA AFFECTS MANY young adults because they spend more time keeping busy than paying attention to their bodies' needs. Blood loss during menstruation puts women at a greater risk of developing anemia.

- The most common symptoms of iron-deficiency anemia are fatigue, exhaustion, breathlessness after exertion, brittle nails, low attention span, headaches, gastrointestinal upset, pale skin, rapid pulse, and loss of sexual interest and desire.
  - ■ Usually a lack of iron is brought on by a diet heavy in processed foods, which are low in all essential nutrients, including iron.
    - * Iron, protein, and copper make up hemoglobin in red blood cells—the substance which delivers oxygen throughout the body.
  - ■ Eat fresh meat, fish, and poultry because they contain a form of iron called "heme"; almost 40 percent of heme can be absorbed by your body.
  - ■ Eat eggs, dried beans, nuts, and whole grains. They contain a form of iron called "ionic"; about 10 percent of ionic iron can be absorbed by your body.
  - ■ Studies show that at least 200 to 500 mg of vitamin C daily helps your body absorb iron.
- Megaloblastic anemia is caused when you don't get enough

folic acid, which comes mainly from green, leafy vegetables, and from alfalfa, soybeans, chickpeas, oats, lentils, beans, wheat germ, liver, split peas, wheat, barley, rice, asparagus, green peas, and sunflower seeds.

■ If you cook these vegetables, nuts, and grains, you will lose 65 percent of their folic acid content.[28]

PREMENSTRUAL SYNDROME (PMS) has been a medical mystery for centuries. Only recently have male doctors accepted the fact that PMS is a real disorder that puts women through many physical and emotional symptoms, including anxiety, anti-social behavior, bloating, swollen and sensitive breasts, confusion, cramps, cravings for salty foods or chocolate, crying spells, depression, dizziness, exhaustion, fluid retention (especially in the legs), headaches, irritability, sleeplessness, and mood swings.

- Two major causes of PMS are strict dieting and eating junk foods, both of which stress the body and mind.
  - When you go on a severe diet, you not only lose body fat, you also lose the small amount of fat that your brain uses to create hormones. What occurs is a hormone fluctuation that wreaks havoc with your body and your emotions.
  - If you have PMS, you should limit or eliminate junk foods, refined sugar and sugary foods, salt, caffeine, coffee, chocolate, and carbonated soft drinks from your diet.
  - You need to eat at least 50 grams of protein daily (about two ounces of turkey, chicken, or red meat) while you experience symptoms of PMS.
  - Eat more cereals, fruits, legumes, vegetables, and whole grains.
  - Cut down on sharp cheeses, and eat cottage and cream cheese instead.
  - An effective nutritional weapon during PMS is unsweetened yogurt blended with a small amount of brewer's yeast, which contains glutamic acid, food for the

brain.

- Eat more potassium-rich foods (bananas, cantaloupe, parsley, peas, avocados, potatoes, cabbage, almonds, peanuts, pecans, sunflower and sesame seeds, and lentils).
- Low blood sugar (hypoglycemia) is a major contributor to PMS.
  - Eating a mid-morning snack of wheat or bran in milk will satisfy hunger and increase the amount of fiber and calcium in your system.
  - Eat six small meals a day instead of three large ones.
  - Take in extra magnesium in foods or supplements.
    * Magnesium releases retained fluids and decreases the desire for chocolate.
    * A 50 mg supplement of vitamin B6 will help your body absorb the increased magnesium.
- Take two capsules of Evening Primrose Oil three times daily.
- Zinc and vitamin E supplements may lessen cramping.
- Regular vigorous exercise will help.[29]

FIBROCYSTIC DISEASE (NON-CANCEROUS lumps in the breast) can usually be stopped and, in most cases, reversed.

- Fibrocystic disease usually comes in three stages.
  - Premenstrual swelling of the breasts that is accompanied by pain and tenderness and usually subsides after menstruation, comes in the late teens and early 20s.
  - In your late 20s or 30s, a number of small nodes may develop in your breasts, often accompanied with a large lump that is easily mistaken for cancer (fibrocystic masses are two-dimensional [high and wide], rather than three-dimensional like cancer).
  - The final stage occurs in the mid-30s and is called full-blown fibrocystic breast disease. Many cysts have formed in the breasts and block the milk ducts, causing a dull pain, a feeling of being milk-filled, and a burning sensation. Occasionally the breast and nipples sting, and

a watery discharge will come from the nipples.

- To prevent or treat this disease, you must stop eating and drinking foods containing chemicals called methylxanthines, which are caffeine in coffee, chocolate, cola drinks, and some tea; theophylline in tea; and theobromine in chocolate.
- A high-fat diet contributes to the disease because fat increases estrogen production, which in turn increases cell production in your breasts.
  - Reducing the fat in your diet will lower your estrogen levels and, therefore, the possibility of developing fibrocystic disease.
- Take 200 to 300 mg of vitamin E daily; and eat more foods with selenium (corn, cabbage, whole wheat, beans, and peas).
  - This regime may also be helpful in preventing and fighting breast cancer.[30]

YEAST INFECTIONS ARE more common in women, but they also attack men because the infection, called *candida albicans*, is caused by a fungus present in every human being.

- Everyone carries small amounts of the candida fungus in the warm, moist areas of the body—the anus, intestines, nose, throat, and vagina.
- The infection occurs when there is an overabundance of the fungus.
  - Symptoms of the illness include feeling drained by fatigue, inability to sleep, poor memory, aching muscles, abdominal discomfort or pain, pain and/or swelling of the joints, premenstrual syndrome, and more.
  - Get a diagnosis from your doctor.
- Yeast infections are not caused by eating too much yeast, but by taking in too much refined carbohydrates (mainly sugar).
  - You can prevent or cut down on the occurrences of the infection by cutting out all refined flour, all types of sugar (white, brown, golden, corn syrup, honey, maple syrup,

molasses and sorghum), all processed foods, and sweetened soft drinks.
- If you have numerous or severe yeast infections, you may have to cut out fresh, frozen, dried, and canned fruits.
- Eat more protein, complex carbohydrates, and yogurt, and only a little fat.
- Take garlic supplements, a multiple vitamin with minerals, a 50 mg table of vitamin B-complex, 1,000 mg of vitamin C, and two cups of Taheebo tea (available at health food stores) daily.[31]

NUTRITION VS. THE AGING PROCESS

Do you take aging for granted? You know you're growing older, so you assume that you are getting weaker and becoming more prone to a variety of illnesses such as cancer, diabetes, cataracts, and senility. But if you believe the Word of God, you know that illness is not an inevitable part of old age. God doesn't want you ill and weak; He wants you strong and powerful, able to carry His good news to the world.

I am in my 60s. I travel all over the world. I spend hours studying the Word; taping my television show; and teaching the Word at Encounters, conventions, church services, and Bible college classes. How do I manage all this? I read and speak the Word, claim God's promises of health and vitality, and follow God's guidelines for living.

We should all live in perfect health. If you lack energy (no matter if you are 70 years old or 30 years old), something is wrong. From the day you're born until the day you die, your body should be exercised and receive the proper amount of nutrition from healthful, natural foods. Don't pollute your body with alcohol, cigarettes, white sugar, white flour, overeating, and overindulgence. You should eat a diet that is low in fat and red meats and rich in raw fruit and vegetables. No matter your physical limitations, you should take part in some kind of vigorous, aerobic exercise. And finally, supplement your diet with vitamins and minerals.

MIDDLE AGE

I want to destroy the myth that says being middle aged means love handles, pot bellies, and flabby arms are inevitable. These things will happen ONLY if you eat the same amount and kinds of food you did as a child and young adult without getting as much exercise.

It's not middle age that determines body fat levels—it is the decreasing number of hours that you devote to aerobic exercise. If you are unable to exercise due to physical limitations, then you should not have to eat as much. However, if you exercise 20 to 30 minutes a day (vigorous, aerobic activity) you will burn your food at the same rate as you did when you were 30 years old.[1]

It's true that your body is not as limber as it was when you were young; however, bodies that have been exercised from childhood through adulthood will be stronger and more limber. If you are able to exercise, then you must! Even if you're 50 years old, it's not too late to begin an exercise program. Just start slowly, stick with it, and pray for strength of body and of will (see YOUR FOOD ATTITUDES).

MATURITY ONSET DIABETES (Type II Diabetes) usually affects people who are 40 years old or older because they have maintained a lifestyle of eating too much (mainly processed foods) and being overweight. The insulin-producing cells in your pancreas function, but the output of insulin is inadequate for your body's needs.[2]

- You may be able to control this form of diabetes (even to the point of not having to take insulin injections) by eating a well-balanced diet.
  - Do not eat sugar, candy, cake, jam, or sugar-sweetened drinks; and do not smoke.
  - Because insulin needs tiny amounts of chromium to escort glucose through cell walls, eat foods rich in chromium (thyme, black pepper, whole wheat, cloves, seaweeds, brewer's yeast, corn oil, vegetables, fruit, honey, chicken, blackstrap molasses, parsley, butter, nuts, grains, maple syrup, eggs, and brown rice).
  - A high-fiber diet helps reduce fat and the need for insulin.
    * Outstanding fiber foods are almonds, apples, blackberries, broccoli, corn, fresh peas, kidney beans, plums, potatoes, prunes, raisins, spinach, sweet potatoes, whole wheat bread, and zucchini.

■ A cup of cooked navy or pinto beans daily slashes the need for insulin injections by about 38 percent.

    * Beans slow down any rise of blood sugar in the body so less insulin is needed. They also help produce more insulin receptors on cells, giving insulin a better ability to rid extra sugar from your body.

• Daily aerobic exercise will also help control diabetes.[3]

STOMACH ULCERS—NOT uncommon to people in their middle years—are open sores on the lining of the stomach or duodenum (the beginning of the small intestine) that are caused by stomach acid and pepsin (an enzyme which breaks down protein) that attack the stomach and intestinal lining when there isn't enough mucus for insulation.

• If you have an ulcer, you probably have stomach or intestinal discomfort, bloating, or pain. If you have black, sticky stools or red, blood-stained bowel movements, you may have a bleeding ulcer and you should see a doctor **immediately.**

• Cabbage juice, tropical bananas called plantains, essential fatty acids from cold-pressed vegetable oils (safflower, sesame, sunflower seed, and soy), whole grain bread and cereals, and the juice of the aloe vera plant may help prevent and even heal ulcers.

• Cut out sources of stress or learn to manage your stress better.

• Do not try to mask stomach pain with antacids. Long-term and continued stomach pain and heartburn may be symptoms of other problems besides gas, including ulcers, angina, throat cancer, and more.[4]

WRINKLES BEGIN TO show up during your middle years. Although you may consider wrinkles an unavoidable aspect of growing older, wrinkles may actually be a signal to you that your diet is deficient of necessary nutrients.

• When you ingest less than 500 mg of vitamin C a day, you will weaken your skin and cause loose skin and wrinkles.

Take supplements of vitamin C ranging from 500 to 3,000 mg daily.

- Vitamin C strengthens connective tissue, which supports and strengthens the skin in much the same way as chicken wire underlies and strengthens plaster.

- Habitual smokers will have lined and wrinkled skin because smoking one cigarette burns 25 mg of vitamin C.

  - Vitamin C is not storable, so a smoker's connective tissue will cave in.

  - Smoking also narrows arteries and capillaries, limiting the oxygen and nutrients they can deliver to cells and the amount of wastes they can carry off.

- If you have lines at right angles to one another or tiny wrinkles on your lower lip, you aren't getting enough vitamin B2.

  - Get vitamin B2 from liver, royal jelly, alfalfa, bee pollen, almonds, wheat germ, mustard greens, eggs, cheese, millet, chicken, soybeans, and sunflower seeds.

- When you don't ingest enough calcium, many signs of premature aging develop, including wrinkles, arthritis, cataracts, and shriveled sex glands.

  - Take a calcium supplement of 1,200 mg daily.

- Daily doses of vitamin E through food or supplements may help prevent wrinkles brought on by stress and overexposure to the sun.

- Eat plenty of citrus fruits, apricots, cherries, grapes, green peppers, tomatoes, papaya, broccoli, and cantaloupe; and drink tangerine juice to lessen the probability or severity of wrinkles.

- Take a supplement of zinc.[5]

60+

Your older years have as much potential for adventure, love, and fun as your childhood. God's promise for health, prosperity, and wisdom do not have age limits. You should not accept the world's restrictions for your own life; nor should you believe the devil's lies that because you are 60 or older you must become inactive, useless, and alone.

You must take care of yourself by eating correctly and getting enough exercise because people who are 60 years old and older are at risk for nutritional problems.[6] The elderly are the single largest group of Americans who are malnourished. They are not able to absorb the amount of nutrients they need to remain healthy because of physical changes that occur with aging. Making things worse is the fact that when an older person is malnourished, the process occurs gradually so that by the time it is recognized it is a full-blown medical problem rather than a lifestyle issue that can be corrected with some simple steps.[7]

Another concern for older people is that an estimated 50 percent of people 60 years and older take two or more prescription drugs and half of this number take five or more drugs. Taking combinations of prescription drugs can suppress the appetite and the body's ability to absorb and use nutrients.[8] Added to this problem is the fact that nearly 50 percent of America's elderly people live alone on fixed incomes, which may decrease their desire or ability to eat properly.[9]

It's important for you to remain active. Do as much as you can (and for some seniors, that may even mean jogging or vigorous walking). Make sure you eat the proper foods and take supplements. Talk to your doctor about vitamin and mineral supplements because they may counteract the effects of some drugs or cause problems at large doses.

If you are a member of a church, get more involved with different activities and programs. If you aren't a member, join a Bible-teaching,

Holy Spirit-filled church this week! Nothing helps combat loneliness better than joining a family of believers. If you are a shut-in, call your church or a nearby church and ask to be part of a visitation program, and offer your services to make phone calls or stuff envelopes.

Make a decision to do something positive and uplifting with your life—hold Bible studies, visit nursing homes (or the other people in your nursing home); write cards and letters or make phone calls to family members and friends even if they live right next door; learn a new skill; get a part-time job; or volunteer at a hospital, cancer research center, soup kitchen, or YMCA. Whether you are in a wheelchair or are able to get around with ease, you have a great deal to offer your family, church, and community.

A POOR APPETITE must be treated because it can be a symptom of some diseases and a sign of nutritional deficiencies.

- The decline in the number of taste buds on the tongue that occurs with age can diminish appetite as well as take away from food's appeal.
- A poor appetite can be a sign that you don't eat enough foods containing vitamins B1 and B12.
  - Either make a point of eating more of these foods or take supplements.
- The loss or decline of the senses of taste and smell is dangerous because without them you will not be able to detect warning odors such as gas escaping from a stove or heater, fumes from an auto's leaky fuel line, smoke from a fire, or the taste of spoiled food.
  - Combat the problem by taking 50 mg zinc supplements daily.
  - If you eat foods high in beta carotene—red, yellow, orange, and purple vegetables—you may regain your sense of smell.
  - Take vitamin A supplements or eat foods high in the vitamin.

- You may lose your appetite if you take prescription drugs, especially chemotherapy drugs which can bring on nausea and vomiting; drink alcohol, which causes a depletion of vitamin B1, protein, and zinc; or have cirrhosis of the liver, gastritis, hepatitis, ketoacidosis, milk intolerance, and pancreatitis.[10]

ALCOHOL IS A particular problem of the elderly. The central nervous system in older people is more sensitive to alcohol's effects than in younger adults, so drinking will impair your thinking and motor skills faster. Since your metabolism is slower as an older adult, alcohol takes longer to leave your system. As an older adult, your body has about 15 percent less water than when you were younger, so the alcohol will be less diluted and cause more problems. Finally, medications can strengthen alcohol's influence.

- Alcohol problems are harder to recognize in older adults.
  - Since many elderly alcohol abusers live alone, their drinking is less likely to cause run-ins with family, friends, and police.
  - The confusion, disorientation, fatigue, clumsiness, and self-neglect caused by alcohol abuse is often mistaken for signs of aging.
- One out of three elderly alcoholics do not begin to drink heavily until late in life and usually as a response to grief or illness.[11]
- Brains of chronic alcoholics disintegrate as cells die.
- A leading cause of cirrhosis of the liver is abuse of alcohol.
  - Cirrhosis causes the formation of scar tissue which replaces liver cells, reducing circulation and causing the liver to malfunction.
  - Cirrhosis can't be cured, but its progress can be halted by cutting out alcohol and adding protein and B vitamins to your diet.[12]
- Studies have shown that when people eat a diet high in raw foods, they immediately and spontaneously avoid alcohol

and tobacco.

- ■ When chronic alcoholics were given a nutritious diet and nutritional supplements, they were able to stay away from alcohol better than people on high-fat, high-carbohydrate diets.

- People who drink alcohol should stop and should eat foods high in, or take supplements of, vitamins A, B1, B2, B6, B12, C, and E; and the minerals magnesium, selenium, zinc, and calcium.

- Evening Primrose Oil and mixed freeform amino acids should also be taken in pill form daily.[13]

OLDER PEOPLE WHO forget things easily and have a diminished memory often jump to the conclusion that they are heading for senility or have Alzheimer's disease. More than likely, however, they are simply malnourished in vitamins and minerals which help sustain mental functions.

- Declining memory may be a result of a deficiency in vitamins B1 and B12, choline, lecithin and magnesium—as well as low thyroid function, low blood sugar, or long-term stress.

  - ■ Faulty memory, as well as low energy, lack of appetite, and emotional excesses, are all symptoms of vitamin B1 deficiency.

    - * If you eat foods containing refined sugar and flour or other processed foods, drink alcohol regularly, or are addicted to coffee, you are draining your body of vitamin B1.

    - * Supplements of vitamin B1 have brought incredible recoveries for people who were considered senile.

  - ■ A deficiency of vitamin B12 can cause a devastating memory loss and inability to think clearly, as well as depression, confusion, delusions, and hallucinations.

    - * The elderly are particularly prone to vitamin B12 deficiency, which can be treated with injections given by a doctor or supplements.

- The memory center of the brain, the hippocampus, has a special affinity for the mineral magnesium.
  - If you have trouble learning and a sieve-like memory, you may be lacking magnesium, so make sure you eat plenty of foods high in the mineral.[14]

THE INITIAL SYMPTOMS of Alzheimer's disease—forgetting names and addresses—are common in the elderly and are often overlooked. It's not until the failing memory becomes worse—not knowing the way home, forgetting how to perform daily tasks—and other symptoms occur that Alzheimer's has progressed far enough to warrant an opinion from a doctor.

- Added to a steadily deteriorating memory and impaired judgment come changes in personality and temperament—anxiety, nervousness, depression, irritability, and temper flareups.
- The person with Alzheimer's will have difficulty thinking and speaking, and will not be able to control bladder or bowel movements.
- He will also experience weakened, easily-fractured bones and painful arthritis.
- Studies have shown that aluminum accumulated in the brain may be the cause of Alzheimer's, non-specific joint disorders, and childhood hyperactivity.
  - Stay away from the following products if their labels say they contain aluminum: acne medications, antacids, anti-diarrhea products, anti-perspirants and deodorants, cosmetics, douches, feminine hygiene products, hemorrhoid preparations, lipstick, skin creams, lotions, and toothpaste.
  - The following foods may contain high amounts of aluminum: factory-made breads and pastries, baking powders, processed cheese, pickles, salad dressings, table salt, white flour, and fruit juices stored in aluminum containers.

■ Don't use aluminum pots and pans, which give off small amounts of aluminum to food, especially if your city's water supply contains fluoride, which causes aluminum to leach from cookware and be absorbed into food.

■ To reduce accumulated aluminum and possibly prevent Alzheimer's, take supplements of vitamin C (about 1,000 mg), calcium, and magnesium daily.

• The amount of acetylcholine in the brains of Alzheimer's patients is reduced by 90 percent, which may cause memory loss.

■ Failing memory can be boosted with supplements of choline (a nutrient found in soybeans, liver, and egg yolks), which converts into acetylcholine in the brain.[15]

AN ESTIMATED 35 million Americans have one of the two forms of arthritis—rheumatoid and osteoarthritis.

• Osteoarthritis is a wearing-away ailment. Cartilage (gristle) in the joints wastes away and calcium spurs form on surfaces which contact bones. Synovial tissues which hold a lubricating fluid and insulate the contact of bone with joint cavities thicken, making movement difficult and painful. This condition usually occurs in people who put their limbs through unusual uses and stresses, such as overexercise and overweight.

• Rheumatoid arthritis is a chronic, inflammatory disorder bringing stiffness, deformity, and pain to joints and muscles; and is caused when your immune system attacks tissues as if they were a threat to the body.

■ Underlying this type of arthritis is poor digestion and absorption which will cause your body to lose necessary nutrients and cause food to ferment in the intestinal tract and toxins to enter the bloodstream.

■ A peculiar kind of malnutrition afflicts some rheumatoid arthritis patients—a deficiency in folic acid, protein, and zinc.

■ Excessive dietary fat seems to contribute to rheumatoid arthritis.

■ Food allergies also lead to symptoms of rheumatoid arthritis, so cut out those foods to which you are allergic. You may help relieve or eliminate your symptoms.

   * Many food allergies are caused by nightshade plants: eggplant, red and green peppers, Irish potatoes, tomatoes and tobacco; chemical additives, colorings, flavorings, preservatives, and emulsifiers; pesticides, herbicides, and fungicides used on and in many of our growing foods; and other noxious chemicals that pollute our planet.

   * Alcohol, coffee, and cigarettes can also contribute to leaky-gut syndrome (a condition in which food and other contaminants make the intestinal lining more prone to leak partially digested, large food molecules in the bloodstream, creating an allergy to that food).

• The following regimen may help you if you suffer from either type of arthritis: 16 hours daily bedrest; 64 or more ounces of water every day; a well-balanced diet; supplements of calcium, magnesium, and iron; no tobacco, alcohol, or refined carbohydrates (junk food); a gradual decrease of drugs and corticosteroid medications to a level you can tolerate; 2,000 mg of vitamin C; 1,000 IU of vitamin D; and 25,000 IU of vitamin A.[16]

CANCER IS A threat for any age group, especially for elderly adults who spent a lifetime eating too much, eating the wrong things, smoking, and remaining idle.

• Stressors such as radiation, environmental pollution, chemical toxins, overprocessed foods, and overexposure to the sun's radiation contribute greatly to cancer; but people who are nutrition-minded and physically strong are better able to fight off the devastating effects of these carcinogens.

• Make sure your diet is filled with fresh, raw vegetables; fruit, grains, nuts and seeds; and is low in fat and high in fiber. Eat plenty of foods with beta carotene; vitamins A, B-complex, C, D, E, and K; and the minerals selenium, magnesium, calcium, zinc, and potassium.

- ■ All of these nutrients are easily obtainable in a well-balanced diet, but supplementation is not a bad idea (as long as you consult your doctor before starting a new regime).
- • Exercise also makes you stronger and your organs more powerful (cancer is notorious for attacking areas of your body that are the weakest).[17]

CATARACTS ARE A condition primarily of the elderly in which the lens of the eye becomes milky or dark; it results in reduced or shut-off vision.

- • Cataracts develop when proteins in the eye lens are exposed to oxidation and light over the years, allowing protein clusters to form a cloudy mass.
- • Research reveals that the deficiency of vitamins B2, C, and D, and the mineral calcium can contribute to the formation of cataracts.
  - ■ When you take extra vitamin C (about 2,000 to 3,000 mg daily), more of it will be delivered to the eyes and will fight oxidation and the formation of cataracts.[18]

CIRCULATION PROBLEMS ARE a common complaint of the elderly and can cause serious medical disorders—blockage of arteries to the heart and cramping with pain in the chest; obstruction of blood to the heart, causing part of the organ to die; blockage of a blood vessel to the brain; impeded blood flow to the leg; diabetic complications; emphysema; kidney disorders; deterioration of the eye's retina; Parkinson's disease (rigid muscles, muscle weakness, slow movements, and tremors); senility; stroke; and varicose veins.

- • Vitamins C, B6, and E help keep arteries clean so blood can flow freely.
  - ■ A 1,000 mg supplement of vitamin C daily prevents

blockages in arteries that bring on heart attacks and strokes and lowers blood cholesterol levels.

- ■ A deficiency of vitamin C in the daily diet can lead to the loss of certain chemical compounds in artery linings creating irregularities in the lining and causing plaque to accumulate.
    - * A high intake of vitamin C makes artery linings smooth.
- • Various foods can keep cholesterol and triglycerides (which will clog arteries) under control; these include dietary fibers such as oat bran, olive oil, and raw carrots.
- • Many natural foods or supplements help keep blood from clotting when it isn't supposed to—garlic or liquid garlic, onions, cantaloupe, olive oil and ginger.
- • Exercise will keep arteries and capillaries supple and youthful.
    - ■ Inactive capillaries collapse and cannot provide enough food and oxygen to muscles.[19]
- • Intermittent claudication is a partial blockage of blood circulation in the legs, resulting in increasing pain until you can't walk any farther.
    - ■ Take 300 to 400 IU vitamin E and make an effort to walk every day.
        - * This regime will increase the amount of blood circulated in the leg and permit you to walk farther before being stopped by pain.
        - * Improvement takes three months or more and this regime probably won't cure you, but it will decrease the threat of amputation by 95 percent.[20]

CONSTIPATION IS ONE of the most widespread and unnecessary ailments of the elderly.

- • When food wastes idle in the intestines, you can experience hemorrhoids, varicose veins, appendicitis, or cancer.
    - ■ The longer waste matter is pressed against the tender tissues of the colon, the longer bowel bacteria have to

change normal substances in the stool into cancer-causing chemicals.

- ■ Chronic constipation can cause colon disorders such as pouches in the bowel well where fecal matter can lodge and putrefy; this causes the pouches to swell and inflame.
- To prevent and treat constipation, make sure there's enough fiber in your diet from vegetables, fruits, and bran; discover and eliminate food allergens; eat at least a cup of lactobacillus acidophilus-containing yogurt daily; take 60 mg of folic acid daily; and *exercise.*[21]

A DECLINE IN the immune function is not always caused by old age.

- The effectiveness of the thymus gland, a major part of the immune system, declines sharply by the time you are 14 years old; it continues to waste away slowly throughout your life.
  - ■ You rush the wasting-away process when you deprive your body of necessary nutrients, thereby weakening your immune system to the point that it can't fight off infection or contribute to efficient wound-healing.
  - ■ A zinc supplement will help the thymus gland and the immune system function at the level of individual cells and body fluids—blood as well as lymph—so you can fight infection better.
    - * If you are highly susceptible to infection, you may be deficient in zinc.
  - ■ Vitamin A guards the thymus gland from shrinking under stress and restores it to normal size after the stress is over.
    - * Vitamin A also boosts the immune system by battling infections.
- Vitamin E and selenium increase immune system effectiveness.
- Vitamin C stimulates the production of gamma interferon, a powerful chemical that slows the speed at which viruses can reproduce in the cells and stimulates the efficiency of

macrophages (large white blood cells) to kill foreign materials and infectious organisms.

- Lipotropics encourage the production of antibodies and stimulate the growth and aggressiveness of phagocytes (cells that destroy bacteria, viruses, and abnormal or foreign tissues).
  - Lipotropics are found in beets, soy lecithin, egg yolk, lentils, rice, split peas, wheat germ, and barley.[22]

MOST PEOPLE WHO have hip fractures have osteomalacia, which is a softening of the bones.

- More than 40 percent of elderly people are deficient in vitamin D, which is caused by living exclusively indoors.
  - Sunlight is necessary to form Vitamin D in the skin.
  - Eat vitamin D-rich foods and take cod liver oil.
- Various products and drugs can create a condition similar to a deficiency in vitamin D (and, therefore, cause osteomalacia) even when there is enough of this vitamin— frequent use of laxatives and enemas (which will irritate the intestinal wall); use of the cholesterol-lowering drug cholestryamine for a number of years; and long term use of anti-convulsant drugs.[23]

OSTEOPOROSIS (WEAK, HONEYCOMBED bones) is NOT a normal part of aging because almost 90 percent of the people in their 60s, 70s, and 80s have solid bones.

- Osteoporosis is a condition in which calcium has been robbed from your bones.
  - The disease is partially caused by maintaining a diet low in calcium.
  - Bones are living objects, constantly losing and gaining calcium and other minerals. Keep a balance—don't lose more calcium than you gain.
  - By the time symptoms come, bone degeneration has begun. You become shorter; develop a hump on the back; bones and joints ache like arthritis; and the skin on the

back of your hands becomes translucent.

- Blood tests for calcium are deceiving because your body's first priority is to keep your blood well supplied with calcium. If your diet is low in calcium, your body will steal the mineral from your teeth, bones, and spine. Robbery on a steady basis over a long period can cause the bones to collapse.

  - The teen years is the best time to begin taking extra calcium to insure against osteoporosis after menopause. The skeleton reaches the greatest bone mass in size and density during adolescence.

  - The recommended daily allowance for calcium is 1,200 mg.

- Even if you are taking in enough calcium, you may not have enough vitamin D, which allows calcium to be absorbed and used in your cells.

- Extra estrogen after menopause will help your bones maintain their density and rebuild.

  - Estrogen, however, does carry a threat of causing cancer.

- You MUST exercise to prevent osteoporosis.[24]

Section Nine
SUCCESS STORIES

Has God been speaking to you about making changes in your eating habits? Does it seem overwhelming to try to change everything at once—the shopping, cooking, eating, and exercise patterns you've developed over a lifetime? Friend, God wants you to be healthy; so follow Proverbs 3:5,6,8: *"Trust in the LORD with all thine heart; and lean not unto thine own understanding. In all thy ways acknowledge him, and he shall direct thy paths. It shall be health to thy naval, and marrow to thy bones."*

I want to encourage you with the success stories of others who have submitted their eating habits to the Lord. They had to realize that they couldn't make the necessary changes in their own strength, but God was able and willing to work in those areas they gave to Him.

Karen was overweight even as a child, and grew up amid the cruel taunts of other children. It didn't get easier when she became an adult:

"When I went away to college, I got really heavy. I was more than 40 pounds overweight, and miserable. For years, I tried every diet in the book—sane ones and crazy ones—and the result was always the same: some weight loss, crashing after a time, and ending back where I started or worse. Over all those years, I always dreamed of weighing 110 lbs. Unfortunately that dream would be dashed again and again in a puddle of self-defeat (or more often, a puddle of chocolate).

"When I was 35, I accepted Christ. Those first six months were the most amazingly peaceful and assuring I had ever known. It seemed like I had mountain-moving faith all the time and every prayer I prayed was answered! The first change God wanted to make in me was that I stop drinking. I didn't exactly have a drinking problem (yet), but I was awfully attached to the cocktail hour.

"Through much bargaining and trial and error (like

all the diets I'd been on) I got nowhere, but God's leading to give it up totally was very clear. Finally, one night, I saw my will power was not getting the job done, so I just turned it over to Him to do through me. I immediately received the victory over drinking.

"Then an amazing thing happened. Without ever consciously praying about it, I began to lose weight. I wasn't hungry when I wasn't supposed to be and my eating habits began to change—I started liking things that were good for me more than I used to. Jesus was meeting my needs—whatever had formerly caused me to seek comfort in food was now being resolved in Him.

"Several months later, I got on the scales—I weighed 110 pounds on the nose! By turning my life over to Him, He was giving me the desires of my heart. I was stunned— after all those years of striving, never had anything been so effortless.

"Ten years later, I still weigh 110 (well, most of the time!) I can't say that I'm no longer conscious of watching my weight—I am. But gone is the pain of struggling and never winning. It has become an area of victory in my life, and there is no doubt that Jesus was the answer!"

And Jesus is the answer for your problem, too! You may be thinking, "I don't have a weight problem, Marilyn, I am only a few pounds above my ideal weight!" Yes, but do you have the energy and stamina you need to accomplish everything that God has called you to do? Don't settle for less than the best of health!

No one would have said that Martha was overweight, but she found that God's will for her life was much better than what she had come to tolerate:

"I have always been petite, and had never been overly concerned with a weight problem. However, as I have gotten older, I realized that the weight did not come off as easily as it went on. Three years ago my son and his two young children moved into my home and my life changed. Over seven months I gained about twenty pounds. It just seemed to creep up on me. I noticed my energy level was depleted, and I just did not feel well. I tried dieting, and would be faithful for a few days; then I'd become so hungry, I would undo all the good I had done.

"I felt that a weight problem was not a big thing to God. He must be more interested in my spiritual life than my physical weight problems, so I just did not want to bother Him. However, I happened to pick up a book and found these words on the cover *'The Lord Will Perfect That Which Concerns Me'* (and You) (Psalms 138:8). I read the book and I went to the Lord. I told my heavenly Father that my weight concerned me, and I could not perfect it myself; He would have to. I also told Him I would cooperate with Him.

"That was sixteen months ago, and God has taught me healthy eating habits. No diets, just lots of fresh fruits and vegetables, chicken and fish. I watch my fat intake very carefully. Praise the Lord! I am back into a size 6 and down to 108 lbs. God **will** perfect that which concerns us!"

Shirley knew she was overweight, but she had given in to her circumstances. God showed her that He cared about her health. He also showed her that her physical health was an outgrowth of her attitude:

"My situation was like that of the man described in Proverbs 25:28 (NIV), '... *Like a city whose walls are broken down is a man who lacks self control.'* A city with no walls has no protection from its enemies. My walls were broken down because I lacked self-control. My food choices, and my lack of exercise blossomed my body to over 200 pounds.

"I had always been overweight, but rationalized that

159

it was 'the way God made me,' and I had to accept myself that way. But God showed me that I was in denial; He wanted me to be healthy. I had tried many times to change before realizing that without God's help it was impossible. He showed me that my lifestyle—my attitudes and values about food and exercise—had to change. God gave me a plan of action. I joined a support group to learn about healthy eating and found that it is eating according to God's design. However, my attitudes about when and why I ate could only be dealt with in the spiritual realm. 'Exercise' always had been a four-letter word to me; but to my delight, when I added the 'P' word (prayer), to the 'E' word it was no longer a struggle! Now it's the best time of my day, spent in communion with my Lord.

"I now rejoice that, because of these healthy lifestyle changes, I have reached and am maintaining a normal body weight for my stature. But most of all, I have a tremendous amount of energy and stamina. I can outdo my children and grandchildren with ease. They look on with some disbelief, but mostly admiration, for what God has done in my life."

I would love to have more energy than the children I know. Wouldn't you? And some of us, because of our circumstances, really need an abundance of energy. I travel all the time, and that can be exhausting. It also makes it more difficult to eat right, especially if I am in a foreign country. Peggy often travels with me, and needs the abundant energy and excellent health that only Bible foods can provide. Here is her story:

"I've struggled with weight all my life. Even in junior high school, I was always dieting. A few years ago I reached an all-time high, and it seemed that it wouldn't be long before I reached another all-time high and then another. I was out of control, and I knew it.

"The 'quick-weight-loss' diets were not working for me

anymore. I had failed so many times, I did not have the will power to deprive myself because I knew that I would just put it back on again—so why suffer and delay the inevitable?

"I prayed and asked God to help me. When I analyzed my failures, I realized that I had always set goals for 'too much too fast,' usually because of a deadline such as a vacation. When I did not reach my unrealistic deadlines, I was discouraged; and the defeating cycle would start all over again.

"The circumstances of my life were difficult at that time. I was under a lot of pressure, and I knew that my out-of-control eating was a symptom of much deeper problems. However, I did not wait until I got those other areas in God's control. He worked with me and helped me right where I was. The extra weight I was carrying only made the other situations worse because I felt so awful about myself.

"I made a commitment to lose weight no matter how long it took. I didn't set a target date; I set a pace that would not make me feel deprived and tempted to quit. I began this program with prayer and a new resolution that 'it would take as long as it would take.' I would work on this for the rest of my life, so there was no reason to rush it. I still had to use discipline. I had to learn how to make wise choices in my eating and say 'no' to some things. I have been at this for about three years. I have lost about 90 pounds and am very close to my weight goal. I have been on a regular exercise program for the past 2 years and enjoy it very much.

"My success is based on sensible eating, regular exercise, and depending on God to keep me going when I get discouraged. I travel frequently, and I have had to remain flexible and to adjust what and when I eat to whatever is happening in my life at the time.

"There are still days when I get discouraged and think I'll never make this last five pounds. Then I stop and remember where I've come from and thank God that He is faithful to complete the work He has started not only within me but 'on' me as well."

Like Peggy, many of you have tried lots of different diet programs. Some haven't worked at all, and some helped you to achieve only partial or temporary success. Yet we have found that only God can make the changes in our hearts that are necessary before we can have real victory in the outward aspects of our lives. Some of us have grown up with deep emotional wounds, and have tried to ease the pain temporarily with food. If this has been your experience, Sharon understands your struggle:

"I've had a weight problem for most of my adult life. For years I tried all kinds of diets, from fads to commercial products. Finally the Lord convicted me to stop dieting and trust Him. Since then, He has led me to form my own life-time diet that is low in fat according to His commands in Leviticus. I also walk every day.

"My greatest breakthroughs have not been these outward changes. The real victory has been the emotional healing He has ministered to me regarding my childhood. I had been carrying anger and frustration all my life, which eventually created a wasteland in me. I had used food to try to satisfy the emptiness. When God delivered me from anger and frustration, and gave me peace, I no longer ate to satisfy emotional needs."

Maybe you need that peace that only God can give. Jesus said, *"Peace I leave with you, my peace I give unto you: not as the world giveth, give I unto you. Let not your heart be troubled, neither let it be afraid"* (John 14:27). But when we don't have a personal relationship with Jesus, we don't have peace. We search everywhere for a substitute that will make us feel better, even just for a short time. Some people turn to drugs and alcohol because of emotional pain, but many "good" people who would never touch those things use food to distract themselves from what hurts too much to handle. Lana did, until she met Jesus:

"A few years ago, my weight was at 279 pounds and climbing quickly. I am only five foot two, and I was killing myself with food. Spiritually, I was hard, cold, and miserable. The turning point came on Christmas Eve. I was home alone, with an emptiness in my heart as big as the Grand Canyon. I spoke to God for the first time in twenty years, 'If You are real, please come into my life. Change me, change my heart, or take me home.' A great peace came over me, and I slept the first peaceful sleep I had known in years. My heart started changing, my outlook on life improved, and my weight started falling off.

"I had checked on commercial weight-loss programs and found that I would have to pay over $800 to participate, and I did not find their food very appealing. I prayed about it. I told God I didn't have the money, but I needed to lose weight and I needed to do it safely. He gave me a better solution. I am very careful about my fat intake. I read labels on everything, and if it has more than two grams of fat per 100 calories, I don't eat it. I never eat beef, only fish, chicken, and turkey.

"In two years I have lost 140 pounds and my health has improved. God has done it for me. I still have more weight to lose, but with God's help I will succeed. I also have gained a new heart and an abundance of energy. I have a love for God's Word and a hunger for it instead of food. I eat to stay alive, I do not stay alive to eat. The joy and peace I have are indescribable. Please give God a chance to help you. Only He can fill the emptiness, not food or people. Give Him the burden, only He can carry it and heal those secret places that are so empty."

It is wonderful to see a hunger for God's Word take the place of a hunger for things that never satisfy. God is sufficient to meet every need in our lives. Jesus said, *". . . Man shall not live by bread alone, but by every word that proceedeth out of the mouth of God"* (Matthew 4:4). Kathy also found in God's Word what she needed to change her eating habits:

"After my first child was born, I continued to gain weight. I just couldn't control my eating habits. I loved chocolate, and eventually developed a compulsion to eat M & M candies that became as strong as, perhaps, the smoking habit is for other people. I began to dislike my looks as I was over 210 pounds and still gaining.

"During a time of intense Bible reading and study, God began to convict me about habits in my life that were not pleasing to Him. One night I couldn't sleep and began to pray. I wept and poured my heart out to God about this weight problem. God showed me that He loves me no matter how heavy or thin I am, but said that He would help me lose weight and get my body back into good condition, if I would commit it to Him.

"God gave me two friends who also wanted to develop self-control in their eating habits. We stood on the verse, *'. . . pray one for another, that ye may be healed . . . .'* (James 5:16). We began to pray for one another! Before I ate anything, I would pray for them. I spent more time in the Word and in prayer, I ate smaller portions, and didn't take seconds. The Lord gave me the ability to stop eating sweets. I ate no sweets at all for several months, until I felt the Lord telling me I could eat some in moderation. Exercise also became important to me, and I began taking daily walks.

"During the next year I lost 40 pounds. God has given me more self-control in my eating habits, but I have discovered I can't lose weight on my own without His direction and guidance. I have tried various diets, but the best, most lasting way for me to lose weight and get my body into shape has been to follow God's plan. I have had to rely on the Lord to change my desires in the area of my eating habits. It has been a complete change of lifestyle. Now I rely totally on the Lord for His strength and guidance; my life is in His hands. '... *My food is to do the will of Him who sent Me, and to accomplish His work*' (John 4:34 NAS). With God's help, I refuse to give in to the temptation to overeat. He has set me free from my former addiction to sweets and overeating. He gives me the self-control, discipline, and wisdom to eat properly. Praise the Lord!"

Kathy learned to rely on God to change her desires. When we trust Him, He will meet every need in our lives. If you have realized that your weight problem is too big for you to handle, that is good news! Because, *"He giveth power to the faint; and to them that have no might he increaseth strength"* (Isaiah 40:29).

Ann was severely affected by an eating disorder that she was unable to solve on her own; she could not even recognize that it existed. The problem was different: a life-threatening weight loss due to anorexia and bulimia. But the solution was the same as all these other women found: trusting Jesus.

"During junior high, I became consumed with my looks. I started intense exercise workouts—5 to 7 hours a day—leading to appetite loss. Eventually I became anorexic and went from 110 to 54 pounds. Even then, I still saw myself as fat.

"My mother began interceding for my healing. In my senior year of high school, I suddenly saw myself as I really looked. At five foot three and 54 pounds, I was a sad sight. I cried out to Jesus to heal my body.

"I saw many doctors who gave me no hope of ever having normal body functions. By this time, I hadn't had a menstrual period for five years because of my low weight. Few doctors believed my body would even partially recover from the damage. But Jesus is a big Savior.

"Through the ministry of the Word of God, Jesus totally restored my body, soul, and spirit. No longer am I consumed with exercise, food, or the compulsion to under- or over-eat. I have a beautiful baby girl, though three doctors said I could never have children.

"Jesus set me free of anorexia, bulimia, and compulsive behavior. He removed the weak places, and even the scars left behind. Freedom through Jesus Christ is the only way to be truly free—body, soul, and spirit."

Did these testimonies inspire and encourage you? Would you like to have more stamina and energy? Just think what you could accomplish! All the plans you have held in your heart for "someday," but could never quite get around to, can be fulfilled.

What is the number-one thing you would do if you had extra energy? If you have been eating the "typical" American diet, and you will make the commitment to follow God's eating plan, you are in for a wonderful surprise. Not only will your weight stabilize at what is right for you, but you will have better health and greater energy. You'll be able to do many things you had only hoped for. You can find the "abundant life" Jesus died on the Cross to give you, when you are willing to live it His way!

Section Ten
RECIPES FOR HEALTHY LIVING
PREFACE

HOW CAN WE make our diet more healthful, and still serve meals our families will be willing to eat? The answer is: gradually! If you toss out all your favorite recipes and serve nothing but tofu, brown rice, and Brussels sprouts, you will most likely find that the dinner table becomes a battlezone. So go slowly! Rather than tell your children that cake and ice cream are gone for good, just begin to serve more nutritious fruit-sweetened desserts occasionally.

Make nutrition an adventure. Most kids don't care for canned peas. But if they are allowed to pick up sliced raw vegetables with their fingers and dip them into a tiny bowl of yogurt-based salad dressing, suddenly food is fun!

If your family includes a meat-and-potatoes traditionalist, you can improve your diet by serving chicken and turkey more often, rather than well-marbled beef. You can still have steak occasionally; just serve smaller portions, and fill everyone up first with a big vegetable salad and whole-grain rolls.

I have some of my personal favorite recipes to share with you, which will give you an idea of how to make changes without making your family feel deprived. Here are some basic tips to modify the recipes you already use:

- Cut back on the serving size of meat dishes. This will only work if you carve the turkey or chicken in the kitchen, and don't put "seconds" on the table. A serving of 3 to 4 ounces per meal is enough for an adult.
- Use lean cuts of meat where possible, and trim fat before cooking. Do not cook poultry in the skin unless you remove it before serving; otherwise, cook chicken or turkey wrapped in foil or covered in a sauce to prevent drying the meat.

- Try not to add fat when cooking. Steam, bake, broil, or stir-fry vegetables; or serve "crudites"—sliced raw vegetables with a flavorful dip. Avoid frying foods. Meat can be baked, roasted, broiled, or barbecued; it can also be stir-fried if it is chopped into very small pieces. Use non-stick cookware and/or a non-stick cooking spray. If you need to add fat, as in sauteing onions and garlic, use a minimal amount of olive oil. If the flavor of olive oil is too strong for a particular dish, try canola oil, safflower oil, or corn oil.

- To remove fat from sauces, soup, etc., chill thoroughly. Fat will float to the top and harden; it can easily be removed before reheating. If you are in a hurry, toss in some ice cubes. The fat will congeal and adhere to the ice cubes. You can remove them, and quickly reheat the sauce if necessary.

- Use vegetable oil in baking, rather than shortening or butter, wherever possible. Sometimes you can substitute applesauce, mashed ripe banana, or crushed pineapple to a recipe and do without oil altogether. For a less sweet taste, try grated carrots or zucchini to replace oil in dinner breads.

- Instead of sour-cream, use non-fat or low-fat yogurt, or puree low-fat cottage cheese in a blender. Spread on baked potato and sprinkle with chopped green onion, or use as a base for dips.

- To use yogurt in cooking, blend in 1 tablespoon of cornstarch or 1-1/2 tablespoons of flour before combining with other ingredients. Cook slowly at a low temperature or the yogurt may curdle. To thicken yogurt without changing the flavor, you can drain it overnight. Line your strainer or colander with cheesecloth or several coffee filters and drain in the refrigerator over a shallow bowl.

- As a substitute for gravy, blend 1/4 to 1/3 cup non-fat dry milk into 1 cup of chicken or beef stock. Be sure to chill the stock first, and skim off the fat. A few tablespoons of non-alcoholic cooking sherry or cooking wine will give it a special flavor.

- Reducing sugar by 1/3 in most recipes will make them more healthful without sacrificing flavor. If you gradually cut back on the amount of sugar you use, your family will become accustomed to the change. Boost flavor with spices such as cinnamon, nutmeg, and allspice, or by adding extra vanilla extract. Almond, lemon, and orange extracts are also available and are a good way to flavor your baked goods. Although honey is better than sugar, it still must be used in moderation. Try sweetening foods with fruit such as raisins, dates, or bananas.
- When you shop for canned fruit, select those packed in water or juice, rather than heavy syrup.
- Substitute whole wheat pastry flour for white flour. Regular whole wheat flour is much heavier than white flour, so it cannot be substituted evenly; for each cup of white flour called for in a recipe, use 7/8 cup whole wheat flour.
- Add oatmeal, oat bran, wheat bran, or wheat germ in small amounts (1 or 2 tablespoons) to cereal, casseroles, baked goods, pancakes, and waffles.

VEGETABLES

TANGY CAULIFLOWER

1 medium cauliflower head, cut in 1-inch florets
2 teaspoons fresh lemon juice
1 tablespoon olive oil
salt and pepper to taste

Cut the cauliflower into 1 inch florets. Steam for 7 to 10 minutes or until crisp-tender. Chop coarsely. Stir in remaining ingredients.

MARILYN'S FAVORITE GREEN BEANS

1 pound green beans, trimmed and cut in half
2 tablespoons butter
1/2 tablespoon olive oil
1 teaspoon minced green onion
1 tablespoon dry vegetable broth (or 1 vegetable bouillon cube)
1 tablespoon fresh (or 1/8 tsp. dried) oregano
1 teaspoon fresh (or 1/8 tsp. dried) thyme
2 fresh sage leaves (or 1/4 tsp. dried sage)
2 cups water

Melt butter in heavy skillet, add oil. Saute onion briefly. Add green beans and saute. Stir frequently and do not allow to brown. Dilute dry vegetable broth in water and run over bean mixture; cover with oregano, thyme, and sage. Bring to a boil, then cover and reduce heat (simmer) for 20 minutes or until beans are tender. Serve with mashed potatoes or pasta, pouring the liquid from the beans as a sauce for the potatoes or pasta.

MARILYN'S FAVORITE HERBED POTATOES

2 pounds tiny new potatoes
1 tablespoon olive oil
3 tablespoons butter, chopped in small cubes
salt and pepper to taste
2 teaspoons fresh oregano, chopped fine
1/2 teaspoon fresh rosemary, chopped fine

Scrub potatoes. Steam potatoes for 20-25 minutes or until tender. Cool to the touch and cut in half. Add 3 tablespoons butter, oil, salt, pepper, and half the herbs and mix. Bake in a preheated 425 degree oven for 15 minutes. Stir well. Reduce heat to 300 and bake 20 minutes longer. Remove from the oven, add remaining butter and herbs and stir.

MARILYN'S FAVORITE POTATO SALAD

6 new potatoes
1 tablespoon lemon juice
6 tablespoons olive oil
1 teaspoon Dijon mustard
salt or other seasoning to taste
2 tablespoons fresh oregano, chopped fine

Scrub potatoes. Steam in covered pan for 30 minutes or until soft. Cool slightly and slice 1/4-inch thick. Combine olive oil and lemon juice and pour over potatoes. Sprinkle with salt and oregano, add mustard, and toss. Can be served cold, at room temperature, or warm. Serves 4.

ORIENTAL BROCCOLI TOSS

2 bunches broccoli
2 or 3 cloves garlic
2 tablespoons safflower oil
1/2 cup vegetable broth
2 tablespoons light soy sauce
1 tablespoon dark soy sauce
2 teaspoons mirin (Japanese rice sweetener) or 1 teaspoon honey
1 teaspoon roasted sesame oil
2 tablespoons cornstarch
1/3 cup water

Trim broccoli florets from stalks. Cut top 2 inches of stalks and florets in 2 inch thick pieces. (Save heavier parts of stalks for other uses.) Steam for 3 minutes. Cool.

Dissolve cornstarch in 1/3 cup water and add 1 teaspoon safflower oil.

Preheat wok or non-stick skillet. Crush garlic, mix with 1 tablespoon safflower oil. In a separate bowl, mix together broth, soy sauces, sesame oil, and mirin. Set both bowls and cornstarch mixture near wok.

Heat 1 tablespoon safflower oil in wok; coat sides. Add garlic and oil mixture; immediately add broccoli. Stir-fry, stirring constantly to prevent burning, until broccoli is coated with oil. Add soy sauce and cornstarch mixtures and toss well. Serves 4.

EASY STEAMED VEGETABLE MEDLEY

2 medium zucchini
2 medium carrots
2 yellow squash
2 summer squash
2 large potatoes
5 tablespoons olive oil

Scrub potatoes and cut in quarters (or sixths if potatoes are very large). Scrub carrots and cut in quarters. Place whole squash and zucchini in steamer with cut vegetables. Steam, covered, for 20 minutes or until all vegetables are tender. Peel potatoes; cut them (and other vegetables) into bite-sized pieces. Add olive oil and salt to taste, toss well.

MARILYN'S FAVORITE ZUCCHINI STIR-FRY

6 medium zucchini, sliced diagonally 1/4 inch thick
2 tablespoons safflower oil
1 teaspoon roasted sesame oil
1 clove garlic
2 teaspoons mirin (Japanese rice sweetener) or honey
2 tablespoons light soy sauce
1 tablespoon cornstarch
1/4 cup water
1/2 cup vegetable broth

Preheat wok or non-stick skillet. Dissolve cornstarch in water. Crush garlic and stir into 1 tablespoon safflower oil. Mix vegetable broth, soy sauce, sesame oil, and mirin. Heat 1 tablespoon safflower oil in wok; coat sides. Add garlic and oil blend and immediately add zucchini. Toss while cooking. Do not brown garlic. Sprinkle with broth if it begins to scorch. Continue heating until zucchini is bright green and slightly tender. Add broth mixture and stir. Add cornstarch and toss well—sauce will thicken. Serves 4.

BREAKFAST DISHES

MUENSTER PIE

1 cup skim milk
1/2 teaspoon salt
3/4 cup flour
1 egg
1 cup shredded muenster cheese
1/8 teaspoon pepper
onion powder, garlic powder, and cayenne pepper to taste

Beat together 1/2 cup cheese and remaining ingredients. Bake in a pie pan at 425 degrees for 30 minutes. Sprinkle 1/2 cup additional muenster cheese on top. Melt in oven for 2 minutes. Serves 4.

MAUREEN SALAMAN'S OAT PANCAKES

1 cup rolled oats
2/3 cup buttermilk
2 tablespoons wheat germ
2 tablespoons bran
1/2 teaspoon baking soda

Combine all ingredients in medium bowl. Allow oats to absorb most of the milk (about 2 minutes). Shape into eight small patties and bake on hot, lightly oiled skillet, turning when browned. Serves 2.

FRUITY FRENCH TOAST

4 slices cinnamon-raisin bread
1 ripe banana, peeled
2 teaspoons frozen orange-juice concentrate
1/4 cup skim milk
2 large egg whites
1/4 cup low-fat yogurt
1 1/2 tablespoons maple syrup or honey
1 teaspoon butter

Mash banana with fork. Stir in orange-juice concentrate. Spread mixture over 2 slices of bread and top with the remaining 2 slices of bread (forming sandwiches). In a flat, shallow dish whisk together egg-whites and milk. Add bread and soak, turning, for 20 seconds each side.

Melt 1/2 teaspoon butter in non-stick skillet over low heat. Brown sandwiches in butter, 5 to 7 minutes. Add remaining butter to brown the other side. Serve with mixture of yogurt and maple syrup. Serves 2.

MAUREEN SALAMAN'S CASHEW-OAT WAFFLES

1 3/4 cups old fashioned oats
2 1/2 cups water
1/3 cup raw cashews
2 tablespoons wheat germ
1/2 teaspoon sea salt

Blend all ingredients until smooth. Bake in preheated medium hot waffle iron 10 to 12 minutes. Do not open before time is up.

GRANOLA

2 cups old fashioned rolled oats
1 cup rolled wheat
1/4 cup soy flour (as a substitute, you can mix 1/4 cup whole wheat flour and 1/8 cup soy grits)
1/4 cup water
1/4 cup canola oil
1/4 cup honey
3 tablespoons brown sugar
1/4 cup wheat germ
1/2 teaspoon vanilla
1/8 teaspoon salt
1/3 cup walnuts
1/4 cup sesame seeds
1/4 cup sunflower kernels

Heat liquids, add brown sugar and salt. Mix well. Combine with dry ingredients. Add nuts. Spread in a low, flat pan and bake 20 minutes at 325 degrees.

MAUREEN SALAMAN'S PUMPKIN PANCAKES

1 1/3 cup whole raw, certified milk
1/2 cup plain yogurt
2 eggs, well beaten
1 tablespoon sesame oil
2 cups whole wheat flour
1 tablespoon wheat germ
1 tablespoon unsulphured molasses
3 tablespoons sunflower seeds, finely chopped
1 1/2 cup pumpkin, cooked and mashed
1/4 teaspoon nutmeg
1/2 teaspoon cinnamon

Combine milk, yogurt, eggs, oil, and molasses. Gently stir in flour, wheat germ, and sunflower seeds. Fold in pumpkin, nutmeg, and cinnamon. Stir until mixed. Spoon onto hot greased griddle. Yield: 10-16 pancakes.

MAIN DISHES

MAUREEN SALAMAN'S LAMB WITH LENTILS

1 pound lamb shank
garlic
3 tablespoons olive oil
1 onion, minced
1/2 teaspoon rosemary
dash cayenne pepper
2 1/2 cups dried lentils
1/4 cup chopped parsley
4 leeks, minced

Cut lamb into 1/2-inch cubes. Insert a garlic sliver into each cube and brown them in 2 tablespoons oil; then add 1/2 cup water and simmer, turning cubes often and adding more water, if necessary, until meat is tender.

Saute onion in 1 tablespoon oil until translucent. Add rosemary and cayenne and bring to a boil. Add washed and strained lentils and 3 cups water. Return to boil, cover and simmer 45 minutes to 1 hour. Stir parsley and leeks into cooked lentils. Divide lentil mixture into 4 servings and top them with equal amounts of lamb cubes.

BAKED RED SNAPPER

1 whole Red Snapper (about 4 pounds), cleaned and scaled
1 lemon, sliced
1/3 cup lemon juice
2 tablespoons lime juice
2 tablespoons olive oil
3 cloves garlic, minced
salt and pepper to taste

Marinade
Beat together lemon juice, lime juice, olive oil, and garlic.

Sauce
4 medium potatoes
1 1/2 teaspoon olive oil
1 small onion
1/2 green bell pepper
3 cans whole tomatoes
1/2 cup non-alcoholic dry white wine
2 tablespoons chopped black olives
1 1/2 teaspoons chopped fresh oregano
dash cayenne pepper
1/4 cup chopped parsley

Slice lemon 1/3 inch thick. Rinse fish; pat dry with paper towels. Sprinkle inside and out with salt and pepper. Cut three deep slashes through to the bone. Insert a lemon slice in each slash. Pour marinade over fish and rub into skin. Cover. Chill for 1 to 2 hours.

Preheat oven to 400 degrees. Lightly grease large shallow baking pan with olive oil or nonstick cooking spray. Peel potatoes and slice thin. Lay potato slices in the bottom of the pan. Sprinkle with salt and pepper. Place fish on top of potatoes. Pour marinade over the fish. Cover loosely with aluminum foil. Roast for 20 minutes. Remove foil and roast until potatoes are soft and fish flesh is opaque (20 to 30 minutes longer).

While fish is roasting, saute onion and bell peppers in olive oil until softened. Do not brown. Add tomatoes, non-alcoholic wine, black olives, and oregano. Simmer 10 minutes, or until most of the liquid has evaporated. Add cayenne pepper and stir well.

Remove fish from the oven. Slide it onto a warmed platter. Arrange the potatoes around the fish. Garnish with parsley. Serve the sauce in a separate bowl. Serves 6.

MARILYN'S FAVORITE BROCCOLI-CHICKEN SALAD

2 whole chicken breasts
2 cups broccoli florets
1 onion
1 clove garlic
1/2 cup parsley
2 cups vegetable broth
1/2 cup low-fat French dressing
1 sprig fresh rosemary (or 1/8 teaspoon dried rosemary)

Halve chicken breasts. Place in saucepan with broth, garlic, onion, and parsley (liquid must barely cover chicken). Bring to a boil. Reduce heat and cover. Simmer for 20 minutes or until chicken is tender.

Add rosemary to water. Use rosemary water to steam broccoli for 5 minutes or until it is bright green and slightly tender.

Remove chicken from bones and chop into 1 inch pieces. Add broccoli, dressing, and toss. Season with freshly ground white pepper to taste. Serve chilled or warm. Serves 4.

SPINACH ROLLUPS

Filling
1 10-ounce package frozen spinach (thawed, dried, and chopped fine)
15 ounces low-fat ricotta cheese (or non-fat, small-curd cottage cheese)
1/2 cup shredded mozzarella cheese
1/2 cup onion, finely chopped
2 cloves chopped garlic
1/4 teaspoon onion powder
1/4 teaspoon garlic powder
1 teaspoon dry parsley
1 teaspoon salt
1/4 teaspoon pepper
2 teaspoons dried basil
2 eggs
1 tablespoon olive oil
1 pound cooked ground turkey (optional)
1/2 cup Parmesan cheese
1 box curly-edged lasagna noodles

White Sauce
1/4 cup butter
1/4 cup flour
4 cups milk
2/3 cup Parmesan cheese
1 10-ounce package frozen spinach (thawed, dried, and chopped fine)
3 cloves crushed garlic
1/4 cup chopped parsley
2 teaspoons basil
1/2 teaspoon salt
1/2 teaspoon pepper

To make sauce, first melt butter and stir in flour. Cook together. Gradually add milk, stirring until smooth. Boil until mixture thickens, stirring constantly. Add Parmesan, stir until melted. In blender, combine remaining ingredients (except spinach), add to flour mixture. Stir in one package thawed, chopped, and drained spinach.

Filling: Saute onions, garlic, and turkey in olive oil. Cook 16-20 noodles in water with oil and salt. While noodles cool, squeeze second package of spinach dry and chop fine. Combine with other filling ingredients; mix well. Remove noodles from water individually. Lay on flat surface. Spread each noodle with 1/3 cup of filling and roll up. Spread 1/2 cup sauce over the bottom of a baking dish. Stand rollups on edge on the sauce. Spoon remaining sauce over the tops of rollups. Bake for 1 hour at 350 degrees. Serves 4-6.

MAUREEN SALAMAN'S BROILED WHITEFISH WITH LEMON BUTTER SAUCE

2 pounds whitefish fillets
1/4 cup butter, melted
1/4 cup lemon juice
2 tablespoons minced onion
1 tablespoon honey
1 tablespoon chopped parsley
2 teaspoons sea salt
dash pepper
6 lemon wedges for garnish

Preheat broiler. Place fillets in broiler pan, skin side down. In a small bowl, combine remaining ingredients, except lemon wedges. Broil fillets 10 minutes, until fish flakes easily when tested with a fork, generously basting fillets with butter mixture. Serve with lemon wedges. Makes 6 to 8 servings.

CHICKEN WITH LEMON-DILL SAUCE

1 pound boned chicken breasts
1 medium green onion
3 tablespoons butter
1 tablespoon fresh dill, chopped
1 tablespoon lemon juice
1/4 teaspoon salt

Remove skin from chicken breasts and cut each into 4 pieces. Thinly slice green onion. Melt butter in large skillet over medium heat. Add onion, lemon juice, salt, and dill. Place chicken in skillet and cover. Cook 10 minutes, basting occasionally. Turn chicken over and cook an additional 10 minutes. Serves 4.

VEGETARIAN MAIN DISHES

MEXICAN RICE CASSEROLE

1 1/2 cups cooked brown rice
1/3 pound Monterey Jack cheese, shredded
1/2 pound low-fat ricotta cheese
1/2 cup cheddar cheese, grated
1 cup cooked black beans
2 3-ounce cans green chiles, chopped
1 large onion, chopped
3 cloves garlic, minced

Mix rice, beans, onion, garlic, and chiles. Layer in an oiled casserole dish, alternating with Jack and ricotta cheeses. End with rice mixture. Bake for 30 minutes at 350 degrees. Sprinkle grated cheddar over the top and return to the oven just long enough to melt the cheese. Serves 4.

CHILES VERDES CON QUESO

2 large ripe green bell peppers
2 large ripe red or yellow bell peppers
4 tomatoes
2 sliced red onions
3 tablespoons olive oil
1/4 cup water
1 1/2 teaspoon salt
8 ounces low-fat cream cheese

Cut peppers in half, remove seeds. Arrange cut-side down on rack and broil 2 to 3 inches from heat until they start to brown. Cut lengthwise into 1/2-inch strips. With a large fork, plunge tomatoes into boiling water for a few seconds; remove and let stand for two minutes. Drain, peel, and chop tomatoes. Saute onions in olive oil. Add peppers, tomatoes, water, and salt. Bring to a boil over moderate heat. Stir in cream cheese and simmer for 10 minutes, stirring occasionally. Serve over steamed brown rice, with corn bread or whole wheat muffins. Serves 4.

MARILYN'S FAVORITE VEGETARIAN LASAGNA

16 ounce can tomatoes
12 ounce can tomato sauce
2 large onions, chopped
1 large carrot, chopped
8 ounce lasagna noodles
6 ounce mushrooms, chopped
6 ounce low-fat or non-fat cottage cheese
5 ounce grated mozzarella cheese
3 ounce grated parmesan cheese
1/2 green bell pepper, chopped
1 large garlic clove, minced
1 tablespoon olive oil
1/2 teaspoon basil
freshly ground pepper to taste
1/2 teaspoon oregano

Saute onions and garlic in olive oil. Add carrot, bell pepper, and mushrooms; continue to saute over high heat to soften vegetables and evaporate liquid. In a large saucepan, combine tomatoes, tomato sauce, oregano, pepper, and basil; simmer for 20 minutes. Cook lasagna noodles according to package directions. Combine vegetables with tomato sauce and simmer another 20 minutes.

Spread 1/4 cup sauce over the bottom of a 12 x 8 inch casserole dish. Place one layer of noodles across the width of the dish. Reserving a small amount of mozzarella, spread noodles with half of cheeses and half of sauce. Add another layer of noodles. Spread with remaining cheeses and sauce. Then sprinkle with reserved mozzarella. Bake at 375 degrees for 30 minutes.

MAUREEN SALAMAN'S LENTIL SOUP

4 cups stock or water
1 cup dried lentils
1 large white onion, diced
2 stalks celery, with tops, chopped
1/2 green bell pepper, diced
2 medium carrots, cut in rounds
1 teaspoon cumin
1 teaspoon nutmeg
1 teaspoon cayenne pepper (optional)
1 teaspoon celery seed
1 teaspoon thyme
1 bay leaf (remove before serving)
1 teaspoon sweet basil
1 tablespoon tamari
3 sprigs parsley, for garnish

Soak lentils for 2 hours (or overnight). To retain maximum vitamins, minerals, and enzymes, cook in soaking water. (To avoid gas, drain soaking water and cook in fresh water.) Bring liquid to a boil and add lentils. Reduce heat and simmer for 30 minutes, partially covered. Add remaining ingredients and simmer for 20 minutes—add 1 tablespoon of tamari last to preserve its nutritional content. Remove half of soup from pan to blender and puree. Mix back into remaining soup in pot. Stir to desired consistency. Top with minced parsley.

WHOLESOME VEGETARIAN SANDWICH

1 whole-wheat tortilla, chapati, or pita
1 cup broccoli
1/2 cup lettuce, finely chopped
1/2 cup alfalfa sprouts, rinsed
1/2 cup cauliflower
3 thin slices dill pickle
2 slices avocado
2 tablespoons yellow squash, finely grated
2 tablespoons carrot, finely grated
2 tablespoons red cabbage, finely grated
1 tablespoon mayonnaise
salt or salt-free seasoning to taste
1/4 cup barbecued onions

Thinly slice broccoli florets and tender upper stalks. Break cauliflower into florets. Steam broccoli and cauliflower for 5 minutes, or until tender. Blend together carrot, cabbage, and squash; mix with steamed vegetables.

Barbecued onions
2 teaspoons safflower oil
1 small white onion
1/2 tablespoon prepared barbecue sauce

Slice onion. Saute in oil. Mix with barbecue sauce.
To assemble: Spread mayonnaise over tortilla. Arrange vegetables and avocado evenly. Spread onions, alfalfa sprouts, and lettuce over the top. Garnish with pickle. Serves 1.

SOUTH-OF-THE-BORDER SANDWICH

8 whole-wheat tortillas
4 cups finely chopped red leaf lettuce
4 cups finely chopped iceberg lettuce
3 cups steamed corn
1 cup chopped tomato
1 cup alfalfa sprouts
1/2 cup steamed, chopped broccoli
3 tablespoons reduced fat mayonnaise
3 tablespoons barbecue sauce
1 tablespoon lemon juice
2 tablespoons olive oil

Combine barbecue sauce, mayonnaise, oil and lemon juice. Mix vegetables together, add sauce and toss well. Heat tortillas; fill with vegetable mixture. Fold up bottom to catch drips and roll. Serves 8.

MARILYN'S FAVORITE AVOTILLAS

6 corn tortillas
reduced-fat mayonnaise
avocado slices
alfalfa sprouts and/or shredded lettuce
seasoning salt or salt-free substitute

Heat tortillas in dry skillet until they are soft but not crisp. Spread with mayonnaise. Place 2 slices of avocado in the center. Sprinkle with seasoning salt (or salt-free substitute). Add a layer of alfalfa sprouts and/or lettuce. Roll up. Serves 2.

LETTUCE "TACOS"

1 tomato
1 bell pepper
1 carrot
1 cucumber
1 stalk of celery
1/2 zucchini
several leaves of lettuce
1 avocado, thinly sliced
alfalfa sprouts

Wash and peel vegetables. Chop finely. Place a slice of avocado in the center of a lettuce leaf. Lay 1/4 cup chopped vegetables over avocado. Top with salad dressing, if preferred. Roll lettuce leaf around vegetables.

MAUREEN SALAMAN'S LENTIL LOAF

2 cups lentils, soaked 2 hours or overnight
1 teaspoon sea salt
tablespoon olive oil
1 medium onion, minced
1 clove garlic, crushed
2 medium peeled, seeded, and chopped tomatoes
2 eggs, beaten

Cook lentils in 4 1/2 cups water with salt for 35 minutes or until done. Heat oven to 350 degrees. Heat olive oil and saute onion until transparent. Add onion and oil to cooked lentils. Add all other ingredients. Place lentil mixture in oiled loaf pan, pat with fork to shape well, and bake for 45 minutes. Good hot or cold.

DESSERTS

LOW-CALORIE CHEESECAKE

4 teaspoons butter or margarine
1/2 cup fine graham cracker crumbs
1 cup low-fat cottage cheese
2 8-ounce packages Neufchatel cheese
3/4 cup sugar
2 tablespoons all-purpose flour
1 1/4 teaspoon vanilla
3 eggs
1 cup and 2 teaspoons skim milk
1 cup fresh strawberries
1/4 cup low-fat yogurt, plain

Melt butter or margarine. Mix with graham cracker crumbs and press into the bottom of an 8-inch springform pan. Beat cottage cheese until smooth. Add Neufchatel cheese, sugar, flour, and 1 teaspoon vanilla; beat together. Add eggs; beat just until mixed. Do not overbeat. Stir in 1/4 cup milk. Fold into prepared pan. Bake 45 minutes in 375 degree oven. Remove from heat and cool 45 minutes. Remove sides of pan; chill cheesecake. Slice strawberries. Arrange on top of cheesecake. Mix yogurt, remaining milk and vanilla together. Drizzle over berries. Serves 12.

CHOCOLATE CHIP BROWNIES

2 cups semi-sweet chocolate chips
1 1/4 cup all-purpose flour
1 cup sugar
1/2 cup unsweetened applesauce
1/3 cup chopped nuts
3 egg whites
2 tablespoons margarine
1 teaspoon vanilla extract
1/4 teaspoon baking soda
1/4 teaspoon salt

Preheat oven to 350 degrees. Melt margarine and 1 cup chocolate chips in double boiler. Add applesauce and sugar, stirring over low heat until smooth. Remove from heat and stir in egg whites. In a separate bowl, mix flour, baking soda, and salt. Stir dry ingredients into chocolate mixture. Add vanilla and mix well. Stir in remaining chocolate chips and chopped nuts. Spread into greased and floured 13 x 9-inch pan. Bake for 16 to 20 minutes or until just set. Cut into 24 squares.

APPLE OATMEAL COOKIES

3 cups quick-cooking oats, dry
2 cups whole wheat flour
1 1/2 cups canned apples, drained
1 cup plumped raisins
(To plump raisins, pour boiling water over them, let them sit 10 minutes, then drain.)
1/2 cup oil
3/4 cup honey
1/4 cup molasses
2 eggs
1/3 cup powdered milk
1/2 cup sesame seeds
2 teaspoons baking powder
1 teaspoon salt
2 teaspoons cinnamon
1/2 teaspoon cloves
1/2 teaspoon nutmeg

Mash apples. Slightly beat eggs. Add oil, honey, and molasses and mix thoroughly. In a separate bowl, combine flour, powdered milk, baking powder, and spices. Add to liquid ingredients and mix. Add oats, raisins, and sesame seeds. Place spoonfuls onto greased cookie sheet. Bake 10 minutes at 350 to 375 degrees.

GREEN APPLE CRISP

8 pippin apples (or more depending on size)
3/4 cup raisins
juice of 1 lemon
2 tablespoons whole wheat flour
1 teaspoon cinnamon
water or apple juice

Topping
Mix together:
1 cup rolled oats
1/2 cup whole wheat flour
1/2 cup brown sugar or honey
1/2 cup margarine or butter
1/3 cup toasted wheat germ
2 teaspoons cinnamon
1/2 teaspoon salt

Preheat oven to 375 degrees. Wash and slice apples. Pour lemon juice over apples, stir to coat. Mix together flour and cinnamon. Add raisins. Sprinkle over apples and stir. Arrange in a greased 9" by 13" baking dish. Pour in enough water or apple juice to cover the bottom of the dish. Mix topping together and sprinkle over apples; press lightly. Bake for 25 minutes, or until apples are soft.

BAKED FRUIT CURRY

1 29-ounce can pear halves
1 16-ounce can apricot halves
1 8-ounce can pineapple chunks
1/4 cup low-fat margarine, melted
1/3 cup brown sugar
1 teaspoon curry powder

Set aside 2 tablespoons of syrup from each can of fruit; drain remaining syrup and discard. Arrange fruit in baking dish. Mix brown sugar, margarine, curry powder, and reserved fruit syrup. Drizzle over fruit. Bake for 20 minutes at 350 degrees, basting occasionally.

BREADS

BARLEY FLOUR MUFFINS

2 cups milk
2 cups barley flour
1/4 cup oil
1/4 cup honey
2 teaspoons baking powder
1/2 teaspoon salt
1/4 teaspoon vanilla extract

Combine honey, oil, milk, and vanilla. In a separate bowl, mix dry ingredients. Fold all together, mixing just until flour is moistened. Spoon into greased or papered muffin cups. Bake at 400 degrees for 20 minutes.

EZEKIEL'S BREAD[1]

8 cups whole wheat flour
4 cups barley flour
2 cups soybean flour
1 1/2 cups warm water
1 cup cooked and mashed lentils
1/2 cup millet flour
1/2 cup warm water
1/4 cup rye flour
1/4 cup oil
5 tablespoons olive oil
2 packages yeast
1 tablespoon salt
1 tablespoon honey

Dissolve yeast in 1/2 cup warm water and let rest for 10 minutes. Mash lentils. Mix with oil and a small amount of water in blender. Then combine with remaining water in large mixing bowl. Combine dry ingredients in a separate bowl. Add two cups mixed flour to lentil/oil mixture and stir. Add yeast. Then stir in remainder of dry ingredients. Place on floured bread board and knead until smooth. Put in oiled bowl. Cover with damp towel and put in a warm place to rise until doubled in bulk. Knead again. Divide dough and shape into four loaves. Place in greased pans and let rise again. Bake at 375 degrees for 45 minutes to one hour. Yields four loaves.

WHOLE WHEAT MUFFINS

2 cups whole wheat flour
1 1/2 cup milk
1/3 cup honey
1 egg, beaten
2 teaspoons baking powder
1/2 teaspoon salt
1/4 cup canola oil
1 teaspoon cinnamon
1/2 teaspoon nutmeg
1/4 teaspoon ground cloves

Mix egg, oil, milk, and honey. In a separate bowl, mix dry ingredients. Fold all together, mixing just until flour is moistened. Spoon into greased or papered muffin cups. Bake for 20 minutes at 400 degrees.

CHILDREN'S FAVORITES

BURRITOS

6 wheat tortillas
1 1/2 cups refried beans
1 cup shredded lettuce
3/4 cup grated cheese
mild salsa

Heat tortillas. Heat beans and spread on tortilla. Sprinkle with grated cheese and lettuce. Drizzle on salsa to taste. Roll up. Serves 4 to 6.

VEGETARIAN SLOPPY JOES

1 onion, chopped
1 carrot, chopped
2 cups lentils, soaked 2 hours or overnight
3 1/2 cups tomato sauce
4 cups stock
3 tablespoons fresh parsley
2 tablespoons olive oil
1 tablespoon tamari
1 clove garlic, minced
1/2 teaspoon basil

Saute onion with garlic in oil until onion is translucent. Add carrot and spices. Simmer for 5 minutes. Add stock and lentils. Simmer for 30 minutes. Add tomato sauce. Continue simmering until lentils and carrot are tender. Serve over lightly toasted whole-grain buns. Serves 6.

MINI SANDWICHES

mini rice cakes
almond butter
honey

Mix equal amount of almond butter and honey (spreads more easily at room temperature). Spread on mini rice cakes. Serve with apple slices and carrot sticks.

PEANUT BUTTER BALLS

3/4 cup natural peanut butter
1/2 cup honey
3/4 cup skim milk powder
1 cup quick-cooking oats, dry
1/4 cup sesame seeds
1 teaspoon vanilla extract
2 tablespoons boiling water
1/4 cup ground nuts

Spread sesame seeds in flat pan and toast lightly in 200 degree oven for 15 to 20 minutes. While seeds are toasting, combine peanut butter, honey, and vanilla. In a separate bowl, blend oatmeal and powdered milk. Gradually add to peanut butter mixture, stirring while blending. When mixture begins to thicken, add 2 tablespoons boiling water and blend. Add toasted sesame seeds. Shape into 1 inch balls. Roll in finely chopped or ground nuts. Makes 36 balls.

SNACKS

MIDDLE-EASTERN SPREAD (Tahini Hummus)

2 cups cooked chick peas
1/2 to 1 cup bean broth or water
2 cloves garlic
6 to 8 tablespoons lemon juice
1/2 cup tahini (sesame seed paste)
1 teaspoon salt

Place all ingredients in blender. Blend to a smooth paste. Thin if desired. Serve as a dip with warmed pita bread.

CHOCOLATE CHIP SNACK SQUARES

1 1/2 cups unsifted all-purpose flour
1 teaspoon baking soda
1/4 teaspoon salt
1/3 cup skim milk
2 large egg whites
2 tablespoons honey
1/3 cup low-fat margarine
1/3 cup frozen orange juice concentrate
1 teaspoon vanilla
1/4 cup chocolate chips

Combine flour, salt, and baking soda. In a separate bowl, mix egg whites, vanilla, honey, milk, margarine, and orange juice concentrate. Stir flour mixture into liquid ingredients and mix well. Stir in chocolate chips. Spread in a greased and floured 8 inch square pan. Bake for 20 to 25 minutes at 350 degrees. Snack squares are done when toothpick inserted in center comes out clean. Cut into 12 squares.

MAUREEN SALAMAN'S DATE-NUT SPREAD

1 cup pitted dates
1/2 cup pistachios
1/4 cup plain yogurt
1/2 cup non-instant dry milk powder

Combine all ingredients in blender. If too thin to spread, add more dry milk powder. Spread on celery stalks.

BLENDER FRUIT DRINK

2 cups freshly squeezed orange juice
1/2 cup plain non-fat yogurt
1 small banana

Whip in blender until smooth. For variety, try using strawberries instead of orange juice, or fresh pineapple juice.

SALADS

ISLAND BREEZES SALAD

2 cups sliced strawberries
2 cups sliced peaches
1 cantaloup, sliced
1/3 cup chopped pecans or walnuts
1/3 cup sunflower seeds
1 1/2 cup unflavored yogurt
1 teaspoon freshly grated ginger
1/4 teaspoon powdered nutmeg
1/4 teaspoon powdered cloves
Honey
Lettuce leaves

Combine strawberries, peaches and cantaloup; mix in nuts and seeds. Stir together yogurt, ginger, nutmeg, and cloves. Sweeten to taste with honey. Fold into fruit mixture. Serve on lettuce leaves.

LEMON YOGURT WALDORF SALAD

1 cup cooked macaroni shapes
3 small apples, cored and chopped
3/4 cup chopped celery
1/2 cup mayonnaise or salad dressing
1/2 cup lemon yogurt
1/4 cup raisins
2 tablespoons sunflower seeds

Combine macaroni, celery, and raisins. Mix together mayonnaise or salad dressing, yogurt, and chopped apples. Spread over macaroni mixture. Sprinkle with sunflower seeds. Chill. Serves 8.

QUICK FRUIT SALAD

2 sliced bananas
2 quartered, sliced apples
2 quartered, sliced oranges
1 pint low-fat, large-curd cottage cheese
1/2 cup chopped almonds
Cinnamon
Lettuce leaves

Mix fruit and nuts together. Stir into cottage cheese. Arrange lettuce leaves on plates; top with mixture. Sprinkle with cinnamon. Serves 4.

Section Eleven
SCRIPTURES FOR HEALTHY LIVING

And God said, Behold, I have given you every herb bearing seed, which is upon the face of all the earth, and every tree, in the which is the fruit of a tree yielding seed; to you it shall be for meat **—Genesis 1:29.**

And God saw every thing that he had made, and, behold, it was very good . . . **—Genesis 1:31.**

Every moving thing that liveth shall be meat for you; even as the green herb have I given you all things. But flesh with the life thereof, which is the blood thereof, shall ye not eat **—Genesis 9:3,4.**

And the LORD spake unto Moses and to Aaron, saying unto them, Speak unto the children of Israel, saying, These are the beasts which ye shall eat among all the beasts that are on the earth. Whatsoever parteth the hoof, and is clovenfooted, and cheweth the cud, among the beasts, that shall ye eat. Nevertheless these shall ye not eat of them that chew the cud, or of them that divide the hoof: as the camel, because he cheweth the cud, but divideth not the hoof, he is unclean unto you. And the coney, because he cheweth the cud, but divideth not the hoof; he is unclean unto you **—Leviticus 11:1-4.**

For it is the life of all flesh; the blood of it is for the life thereof: therefore I said unto the children of Israel, Ye shall eat the blood of no manner of flesh: for the life of all flesh is the blood thereof: whosoever eateth it shall be cut off **—Leviticus 17:14.**

*And he will love thee, and bless thee, and multiply thee: he will also bless the fruit of thy womb, and the fruit of thy land, thy corn, and thy wine, and thine oil, the increase of thy kine, and the flocks of thy sheep, in the land which he sware unto thy fathers to give thee. Thou shalt be blessed above all people: there shall not be male or female barren among you, or among your cattle. And the LORD will take away from thee all sickness, and will put none of the evil diseases of Egypt, which thou knowest, upon thee; but will lay them upon all them that hate thee—***Deuteronomy 7:13-15.***

*When thou hast eaten and art full, then thou shalt bless the LORD thy God for the good land which he hath given thee —***Deuteronomy 8:10.***

*And Elisha died, and they buried him. And the bands of the Moabites invaded the land at the coming in of the year. And it came to pass, as they were burying a man, that, behold, they spied a band of men; and they cast the man into the sepulcher of Elisha: and when the man was let down, and touched the bones of Elisha, he revived, and stood up on his feet—***II Kings 13:20,21.***

*Then he said unto them, Go your way, eat the fat, and drink the sweet, and send portions unto them for whom nothing is prepared: for this day is holy unto our Lord: neither be ye sorry; for the joy of the LORD is your strength—***Nehemiah 8:10.***

*Fear came upon me, and trembling, which made all my bones to shake—***Job 4:14.***

*At destruction and famine thou shalt laugh: neither shalt thou be afraid of the beasts of the earth—***Job 5:22.***

*My soul is weary of my life; I will leave my complaint upon myself; I will speak in the bitterness of my soul—***Job 10:1.***

But thou art holy, O thou that inhabitest the praises of Israel
—**Psalms 22:3.**

Yea, though I walk through the valley of the shadow of death, I will fear no evil: for thou art with me; thy rod and thy staff they comfort me—**Psalms 23:4.**

For his anger endureth but a moment; in his favour is life: weeping may endure for a night, but joy cometh in the morning
—**Psalms 30:5.**

For my life is spent with grief, and my years with sighing: my strength faileth because of mine iniquity, and my bones are consumed—**Psalms 31:10.**

I sought the LORD, and he heard me, and delivered me from all my fears—**Psalms 34:4.**

The wicked plotteth against the just, and gnasheth upon him with his teeth. The LORD shall laugh at him: for he seeth that his day is coming—**Psalms 37:12,13.**

And call upon me in the day of trouble: I will deliver thee, and thou shalt glorify me—**Psalms 50:15.**

What time I am afraid, I will trust in thee—**Psalms 56:3.**

By reason of the voice of my groaning my bones cleave to my skin—**Psalms 102:5.**

He shall not be afraid of evil tidings: his heart is fixed, trusting in the LORD—**Psalms 112:7.**

*In the day when I cried thou answeredst me, and strengthenedst me with strength in my soul—***Psalms 138:3.**

*The fear of the LORD is the beginning of knowledge: but fools despise wisdom and instruction—***Proverbs 1:7.**

*But whoso hearkeneth unto me shall dwell safely, and shall be quiet from fear of evil—***Proverbs 1:33.**

My son, let not them [wisdom, understanding, and knowledge] *depart from thine eyes: keep sound wisdom and discretion: So shall they be life unto thy soul, and grace to thy neck. Then shalt thou walk in thy way safely, and thy foot shall not stumble. When thou liest down, thou shalt not be afraid: yea, thou shalt lie down, and thy sleep shall be sweet—***Proverbs 3:21-24.**

*Keep thy heart with all diligence; for out of it are the issues of life—***Proverbs 4:23.**

*My son, keep thy father's commandment, and forsake not the law of thy mother: Bind them continually upon thine heart, and tie them about thy neck. When thou goest, it shall lead thee; when thou sleepest, it shall keep thee; and when thou awakest, it shall talk with thee—***Proverbs 6:20-22.**

*For by me thy days shall be multiplied, and the years of thy life shall be increased—***Proverbs 9:11.**

*The LORD will not suffer the soul of the righteous to famish: but he casteth away the substance of the wicked—***Proverbs 10:3.**

*The fear of the LORD prolongeth days: but the years of the wicked shall be shortened—***Proverbs 10:27.**

*The merciful man doeth good to his own soul: but he that is cruel troubleth his own flesh—***Proverbs 11:17.**

*A virtuous woman is a crown to her husband: but she that maketh ashamed is as rottenness in his bones—***Proverbs 12:4.**

*A man shall be satisfied with good by the fruit of his mouth: and the recompense of a man's hands shall be rendered unto him. There is that speaketh like the piercings of a sword: but the tongue of the wise is health—***Proverbs 12:14,18.**

*The righteous eateth to the satisfying of his soul: but the belly of the wicked shall want—***Proverbs 13:25.**

*A sound heart is the life of the flesh: but envy the rottenness of the bones—***Proverbs 14:30.**

*A merry heart maketh a cheerful countenance: but by sorrow of the heart the spirit is broken—***Proverbs 15:13.**

*All the days of the afflicted are evil: but he that is of a merry heart hath a continual feast—***Proverbs 15:15.**

*Better is a dinner of herbs where love is, than a stalled ox and hatred therewith—***Proverbs 15:17.**

*The light of the eyes rejoiceth the heart: and a good report maketh the bones fat—***Proverbs 15:30.**

*Pleasant words are as an honeycomb, sweet to the soul, and health to the bones—***Proverbs 16:24.**

*A merry heart doeth good like a medicine: but a broken spirit drieth the bones—***Proverbs 17:22.**

A man's belly shall be satisfied with the fruit of his mouth; and with the increase of his lips shall he be filled—**Proverbs 18:20.**

Slothfulness casteth into a deep sleep; and an idle soul shall suffer hunger—**Proverbs 19:15.**

And put a knife to thy throat, if thou be a man given to appetite. Be not desirous of his dainties: for they are deceitful meat—**Proverbs 23:2,3.**

Be not among winebibbers; among riotous eaters of flesh: For the drunkard and the glutton shall come to poverty: and drowsiness shall clothe a man with rags—**Proverbs 23:20,21.**

Hast thou found honey? eat so much as is sufficient for thee, lest thou be filled therewith, and vomit it—**Proverbs 25:16.**

The north wind driveth away rain: so doth an angry countenance a backbiting tongue—**Proverbs 25:23.**

It is not good to eat much honey: so for men to search their own glory is not glory—**Proverbs 25:27.**

As the bird by wandering, as the swallow by flying, so the curse causeless shall not come—**Proverbs 26:2.**

The full soul loatheth an honeycomb; but to the hungry soul every bitter thing is sweet—**Proverbs 27:7.**

Remove far from me vanity and lies: give me neither poverty nor riches; feed me with food convenient for me—**Proverbs 30:8.**

I know that, whatsoever God doeth, it shall be for ever: nothing can be put to it, nor any thing taken from it: and God doeth it, that men should fear before him—**Ecclesiastes 3:14.**

The sleep of a labouring man is sweet, whether he eat little or much: but the abundance of the rich will not suffer him to sleep—**Ecclesiastes 5:12.**

Behold, God is my salvation; I will trust, and not be afraid: for the LORD JEHOVAH is my strength and my song; he also is become my salvation—**Isaiah 12:2.**

Thou wilt keep him in perfect peace, whose mind is stayed on thee: because he trusteth in thee. Trust ye in the LORD for ever: for in the LORD JEHOVAH is everlasting strength—**Isaiah 26:3,4.**

When the poor and needy seek water, and there is none, and their tongue faileth for thirst, I the LORD will hear them, I the God of Israel will not forsake them—**Isaiah 41:17.**

For I will pour water upon him that is thirsty, and floods upon the dry ground: I will pour my spirit upon thy seed, and my blessing upon thine offspring—**Isaiah 44:3.**

Is not this the fast that I have chosen? to loose the bands of wickedness, to undo the heavy burdens, and to let the oppressed go free, and that ye break every yoke?—**Isaiah 58:6.**

For I will restore health unto thee, and I will heal thee of thy wounds, saith the LORD; because they called thee an Outcast, saying, This is Zion, whom no man seeketh after—**Jeremiah 30:17.**

Take thou also unto thee wheat, and barley, and beans, and lentiles, and millet, and fitches, and put them in one vessel, and make thee bread thereof, according to the number of the days that thou shalt lie upon thy side, three hundred and ninety days shalt thou eat thereof—**Ezekiel 4:9.**

And the king appointed them a daily provision of the king's meat, and of the wine which he drank: so nourishing them three years, that at the end thereof they might stand before the king. But Daniel purposed in his heart that he would not defile himself with the portion of the king's meat, nor with the wine which he drank: therefore he requested of the prince of the eunuchs that he might not defile himself. Prove thy servants, I beseech thee, ten days; and let them give us pulse to eat, and water to drink. Then let our countenance be looked upon before thee, and the countenance of the children that eat of the portion of the king's meat: and as thou seest, deal with thy servants. So he consented to them in this matter, and proved them ten days. And at the end of ten days their countenances appeared fairer and fatter in flesh than all the children which did eat the portion of the king's meat—**Daniel 1:5,8,12-15.**

When I heard, my belly trembled; my lips quivered at the voice: rottenness entered into my bones, and I trembled in myself, that I might rest in the day of trouble: when he cometh up unto the people, he will invade them with his troops—**Habakkuk 3:16.**

For I am the LORD, I change not; therefore ye sons of Jacob are not consumed—**Malachi 3:6.**

But thou, when thou fastest, anoint thine head, and wash thy face; That thou appear not unto men to fast, but unto thy Father which is in secret: and thy Father, which seeth in secret, shall reward thee openly—**Matthew 6:17,18.**

Watch ye and pray, lest ye enter into temptation. The spirit truly is ready, but the flesh is weak—**Mark 14:38.**

And it came to pass, as he sat at meat with them, he took bread, and blessed it, and brake, and gave to them. And their eyes were opened, and they knew him; and he vanished out of their sight —**Luke 24:30,31.**

But as many as received him, to them gave he power to become the sons of God, even to them that believe on his name—**John 1:12.**

For God so loved the world, that he gave his only begotten Son, that whosoever believeth in him should not perish, but have everlasting life—**John 3:16.**

And at midnight Paul and Silas prayed, and sang praises unto God: and the prisoners heard them. And suddenly there was a great earthquake, so that the foundations of the prison were shaken: and immediately all the doors were opened, and every one's bands were loosed—**Acts 16:25,26.**

When he therefore was come up again, and had broken bread, and eaten, and talked a long while, even til break of day, so he departed—**Acts 20:11.**

Wherefore I pray you to take some meat; for this is for your health: for there shall not an hair fall from the head of any of you. And when he had thus spoken, he took bread, and gave thanks to God in presence of them all: and when he had broken it, he began to eat. Then were they all of good cheer, and they also took some meat—**Acts 27:34-36.**

Likewise the Spirit also helpeth our infirmities: for we know not what we should pray for as we ought: but the Spirit itself maketh intercession for us with groanings which cannot be uttered. And he that searcheth the hearts knoweth what is the mind of the Spirit, because he maketh intercession for the saints according to the will of God. And we know that all things work together for good to them that love God, to them who are the called according to his purpose **—Romans 8:26-28.**

For the kingdom of God is not meat and drink; but righteousness, and peace, and joy in the Holy Ghost—**Romans 14:17.**

Whether therefore ye eat, or drink, or whatsoever ye do, do all to the glory of God—**I Corinthians 10:31.**

For I have received of the Lord that which also I delivered unto you, That the Lord Jesus the same night in which he was betrayed took bread: And when he had given thanks, he brake it, and said, Take, eat: this is my body, which is broken for you: this do in remembrance of me—**I Corinthians 11:23,24.**

Casting down imaginations, and every high thing that exalteth itself against the knowledge of God, and bringing into captivity every thought to the obedience of Christ—**II Corinthians 10:5.**

Let all bitterness, and wrath, and anger, and clamour, and evil speaking, be put away from you, with all malice—**Ephesians 4:31.**

I can do all things through Christ which strengtheneth me —**Philippians 4:13.**

Forbidding to marry, and commanding to abstain from meats, which God hath created to be received with thanksgiving of them which believe and know the truth. For every creature of God is good, and nothing to be refused, if it be received with thanksgiving: For it is sanctified by the word of God and prayer—**I Timothy 4:3-5.**

For God hath not given us the spirit of fear; but of power, and of love, and of a sound mind—**II Timothy 1:7.**

Looking diligently lest any man fail of the grace of God; lest any root of bitterness springing up trouble you, and thereby many be defiled—**Hebrews 12:15.**

Submit yourselves therefore to God. Resist the devil, and he will flee from you—**James 4:7.**

If we confess our sins, he is faithful and just to forgive us our sins, and to cleanse us from all unrighteousness—**I John 1:9.**

He that sayeth he is in the light, and hateth his brother, is in darkness even until now—**I John 2:9.**

There is no fear in love; but perfect love casteth out fear: because fear hath torment. He that feareth is not made perfect in love—**I John 4:18.**

Beloved, I wish above all things that thou mayest prosper and be in health, even as thy soul prospereth—**III John 2.**

ENDNOTES

SECTION 1
GUIDELINES FOR HEALTHY EATING
[1]Carlson Wade, The Miracle of Bible Healing Foods, (Boca Raton, FL: Globe Communications Corp., 1991), p. 9.

[2]Stormie Omartian, Greater Health—God's Way: Seven Steps to Health, Youthfulness and Vitality, (Chatsworth, CA: Sparrow Press, 1984), pp. 65,66.

[3]Ibid., pp. 55,56.

[4]Maureen Salaman, The Diet Bible: The Bible For Dieters, (Menlo Park, CA: Statford Publishing Inc., 1990), pp. 6,7.

[5]Ibid., pp. 17,18.

[6]Omartian, op. cit., pp. 58,59.

[7]Salaman, op. cit., p. xvii.

[8]Brian Edmonds, The Doctors' Book of Bible Healing Foods, (Boca Raton, FL: Globe Communications Corp., 1992), p. 21.

[9]Salaman, op. cit., p. 128.

[10]James O'Brien, Super Foods, (Boca Raton, FL: Globe Communications Corp., 1992), p. 6.

[11]Edmonds, op. cit., pp. 6,7.

[12]Ibid., pp. 10,11.

[13]Ibid., pp. 21,22.

[14]O'Brien, op. cit., p. 9.

[15]Edmonds, op. cit., pp. 26,27.

[16]Ibid., p. 27.

[17]Ibid., p. 29.

[18]Ibid., pp. 22,23.

[19]O'Brien, op. cit., p. 13.

[20]Maureen Salaman and James F. Scheer, Foods That Heal, (Menlo Park, CA: Statford Publishing Inc., 1989), pp. 267,268.

[21]Edmonds, op. cit., p. 24.

[22]Ibid., p. 25.

[23]O'Brien, op. cit., p. 20.

[24]Edmonds, op. cit., p. 28.

[25]Salaman (Diet Bible), op. cit., p. 232.

[26]Edmonds, op. cit., pp. 8,9.

[27]Salaman (Diet Bible), loc. cit.

[28]Edmonds, op. cit., pp. 11,12.

[29]Ibid., pp. 12,13.

[30]O'Brien, op. cit., p. 27.

[31]Edmonds, op. cit., pp. 31-33.

[32]O'Brien, op. cit., pp. 27,28.

[33]Edmonds, op. cit., p. 37.

[34]Ibid, pp. 37,38.

[35]Ibid, p. 42.

[36]O'Brien, op. cit., pp. 39,40.

[37]Edmonds, op. cit., pp. 43,44.

[38]O'Brien, op. cit., p. 34.

[39]Edmonds, op. cit., p. 45.

[40]Ibid, pp. 9,10.

[41]Ibid, pp. 47,48.

[42]O'Brien, op. cit., p. 50.

[43]Edmonds, op. cit., pp. 45,46.

[44]Omartian, op. cit., p. 59.

[45]Wade, op. cit., p. 39.

[46]Edmonds, op. cit., pp. 7,8.

[47]Ibid, pp. 13,14.

[48]Ibid, pp. 15,16.

[49]Ibid, pp. 17,18.

[50]O'Brien, op. cit., p. 51.

[51]Edmonds, op. cit., pp. 18,19.

[52]Omartian, op. cit., p. 59.

[53]Edmonds, op. cit., pp. 57-59.

[54]Ibid., p. 19.

[55]O'Brien, op. cit., p. 43.

[56]Omartian, op. cit., pp. 58,59.

[57]Wade, op. cit., p. 53.

[58]Salaman and Scheer (Foods That Heal), op. cit., pp. 165,166.

[59]Salaman (Diet Bible), pp. 58,59.

[60]Ibid., pp. 166-169.

[61]Ibid., pp. 62,63.

[62]Salaman and Scheer (Foods That Heal), op. cit., p. 66.

[63]Salaman (Diet Bible), loc. cit.

[64]Edmonds, op. cit., pp. 61,62.

[65]Ibid., p. 62.

[66]O'Brien, op. cit., p. 59.

[67]Edmonds, op. cit., pp. 60,61.

[68]O'Brien, op. cit., p. 61.

[69]Salaman (Diet Bible), op. cit., p. 203.

[70]Salaman and Scheer (Foods That Heal), op. cit., pp. 367,368.

[71]Ibid., p. 63.

[72]Edmonds, op. cit., pp. 62-64.

[73]O'Brien, op. cit., p. 67.

[74]Edmonds, op. cit., pp. 54,55.

[75]O'Brien, op. cit., p. 62.

[76]Edmonds, op. cit., pp. 55,56.

[77]Omartian, op. cit., pp. 80,81.

[78]Salaman (Diet Bible), op. cit., p. 126.

[79]Salaman and Scheer (Foods That Heal), op. cit., pp. 210,420.

[80]Omartian, loc. cit.

[81]Salaman and Scheer (Foods That Heal), op. cit., pp. 126,127.

[82]Ibid., p. 442.

[83]Ibid., p. 82.

[84]Ibid., p. 38.

[85]Ibid., p. 306.

[86]Ibid., p. 94.

[87]Ibid., p. 86.

[88]Ibid., p. 94.

[89]Ibid., p. 305.

[90]Ibid., p. 81.

[91]Ibid., p. 241.

[92]Ibid., p. 100.

[93]Ibid., p. 132.

[94]Ibid., p. 210.

[95]Salaman (Diet Bible), op. cit., p. 141.

[96]Salaman and Scheer (Foods That Heal), op. cit., p. 209.

[97]Ibid., p. 186.

[98]Ibid., p. 335.

[99]Ibid., p. 388.

[100]Ibid., p. 100.

[101]Ibid., p. 439.

[102]Ibid., p. 276.

SECTION 2
HEALTHY APPETITES FOR A LONG LIFE

[1]Stormie Omartian, Greater Health—God's Way: Seven Steps to Health, Youthfulness and Vitality, (Chatsworth, CA: Sparrow Press, 1984), p. 52.

[2]Ibid., pp. 54,55.

[3]Ibid., p. 52-54.

[4]Ibid, p. 52,53.

[5]Ibid, p. 125.

[6]Ibid, pp. 126,127.

[7]Ibid, pp. 131,132.

[8]Ibid, pp. 130-133.

[9]Maureen Salaman and James F. Scheer, Foods That Heal, (Menlo Park, CA: Statford Publishing Inc., 1989), p. 51.

[10]Omartian, op. cit., pp. 67,68.

[11]Ibid, p. 60.

[12]Ibid, p. 59.

[13]Ibid, p. 56.

[14]Salaman, op. cit., pp. 43-45.

[15]Ibid, pp. 112,113.
[16]Omartian, op. cit., pp. 57,58.
[17]Ibid, p. 61.
[18]Ibid, p. 62.
[19]Ibid, p. 63.
[20]Ibid, pp. 64,65.

SECTION 3
YOUR FOOD ATTITUDES FOR HEALTHY LIVING

[1]Stormie Omartian, Greater Health—God's Way: Seven Steps to Health, Youthfulness and Vitality, (Chatsworth, CA: Sparrow Press, 1984), pp. 67,68.

[2]Maureen Salaman, The Diet Bible: The Bible For Dieters, (Menlo Park, CA: Statford Publishing Inc., 1990), p. 78.

[3]Ibid., pp. 67-71.

[4]Ibid., p. 72.

[5]Maureen Salaman and James F. Scheer, Foods That Heal, (Menlo Park, CA: Statford Publishing Inc., 1989), pp. 214,215.

[6]Ibid., p. 288.

[7]Maureen Salaman, Nutrition: The Cancer Answer, (Menlo Park, CA: Statford Publishing Inc., 1984), pp. 142-144.

[8]Salaman (Diet Bible), op. cit., pp. 74,75.

[9]Ibid., pp. 120,121.

[10]Salaman (Foods That Heal), op. cit., p. 328.

[11]Ibid., p. 334.

[12]Salaman (Diet Bible), op. cit., p. 75.

[13]Ibid.

[14]Ibid., p. 80.

[15]Ibid., p. 23.

[16]Ibid., pp. 16,17.

[17]Ibid., pp. 20,21.

[18]Salaman (Foods That Heal), op. cit., pp. 202,203.

[19]Salaman (Diet Bible), op. cit., p. 21.

[20]Ibid., p. 16.

[21]Omartian, op. cit., p. 67.

[22]Ibid., pp. 75-78.

[23]Ibid., pp. 88,89.

[24]Ibid.

[25]Salaman (Foods That Heal), op. cit., p. 288.

[26]Salaman (Diet Bible), op. cit., p. 55.

[27]Omartian, loc. cit.

[28]Salaman (Foods That Heal), op. cit., p. 177.

[29]Ibid., p. 293.

[30]Ibid., p. 396.

[31]Ibid., pp. 217,218.

[32]Ibid., p. 365.

[33]Ibid., p. 381.

[34]Omartian, op. cit., p. 90.

[35]Ibid., p. 100.

[36]Ibid., p. 104.

[37]Salaman (Foods That Heal), op. cit., p. 177.

[38]Omartian, op. cit., p. 95.

[39]Ibid., p. 93.

[40]Salaman (Diet Bible), op. cit., p. 109.

[41]Omartian, op. cit., p. 96.

[42]Ibid., pp. 97,98.

[43]Ibid.

[44]Laurie Tarkan, "5 Moves That Trim It All," Family Circle, 23 February 1993, pp. 82,83.

[45]Jethro Kloss, Back to Eden, (New York, New York: Lancer Books, Inc., 1971), p. 115.

[46]Omartian, op. cit., pp. 113,114.

[47]Ibid., p. 115.

[48]Ibid., p. 116.

[49]Ibid., pp. 118,119.

SECTION 5
SHEDDING THE HABITS THAT WEIGH YOU DOWN

[1]Stormie Omartian, Greater Health—God's Way: Seven Steps to Health, Youthfulness and Vitality, (Chatsworth, CA: Sparrow Press, 1984), p. 38.

[2]Stormie Omartian, A Step in the Right Direction: Your Guide to Inner Happiness, (Nashville, TN: Thomas Nelson Publishers, 1984), p. 198.

[3]Rocky Mountain News Wire Services, "Study Puts Doctors on Alert for Patients Suffering Depression," Rocky Mountain News [Denver, CO], 12 April 1993, Sec. A, p. 2.

[4]Maureen Salaman, Foods That Heal, Cravings/Addictions, Conquer Cravings For: Chocolate, Alcohol & Tobacco!, (Menlo Park, CA: Maureen Salaman's Nutritional Ministries).

[5]Rocky Mountain News Wire Services, op. cit. p. 24.

[6]Associated Press, "Defining Major Depression," Rocky Mountain News [Denver, CO], 12 April 1993, Sec. A, p. 24.

[7]Salaman (Cravings/Addictions), loc. cit.

[8]Maureen Salaman and James F. Scheer, Foods That Heal, (Menlo Park, CA: Statford Publishing Inc., 1989), pp. 206,209.

[9]Ibid.

[10]Salaman (Cravings/Addictions), loc. cit.

[11]Salaman (Foods That Heal), op. cit., p. 208.

[12]Ibid., p. 206.

[13]Ibid., p. 40.

[14]Salaman (Cravings/Addictions), loc. cit.

[15]Salaman (Foods That Heal), op. cit., p. 40.

[16]Ibid., pp. 207,208.

[17]Ibid., p. 209.

[18]Salaman (Cravings/Addictions), loc. cit.

[19]Ibid.

SECTION 6
CHANGE OF LIFE? MAKE IT A CHANGE FOR THE BETTER!

[1]Gail Sheehy, The Silent Passage Menopause, New York, New York: Random House, Inc., 1991), pp. 1,2,7.

[2]Ibid., pp. 8,23.

[3]Ibid., p. 25.

[4]Ibid., pp. 8,9.

[5]Ibid., p. 9.

[6]Ibid., p. 10.

[7]Ibid., p. 9.

[8]Ibid., p. 12.

[9]Ibid., p. 77.

[10]Ibid., p. 79.

[11]Ibid., pp. 13,14.

[12]Ibid., p. 7.

[13]Ibid., p. 24.

[14]Ibid., pp. 58,59.

[15]Ibid., pp. 24,25.

[16]Ibid., pp. 41,42.

[17]Ibid., p. 25.

[18]Ibid., p. 65.

[19]Ibid., p. 7.

[20]Ibid., pp. 66,67.

[21]Ibid., pp. 81,82.

[22]Ibid., pp. 86,87.

[23]Maureen Salaman and James F. Scheer, Foods That Heal, (Menlo Park, CA: Statford Publishing Inc., 1989), p. 359.

[24]Sheehy, op. cit., pp. 66,67.

[25]Ibid., pp. 106-109.

[26]Ibid., pp. 108-111.

[27]Ibid., pp. 113-115.

[28]Ibid., p. 116.

[29]Ibid., p. 106.

[30]Ibid., p. 122.

[31]Ibid., p. 18.
[32]Ibid., p. 123.
[33]Ibid., p. 127.
[34]Ibid., p. 129.
[35]Ibid., pp. 128-130.
[36]Salaman, op. cit., p. 359.
[37]Sheehy, op. cit., p. 133.

SECTION 7
RAISING HEALTHY KIDS IN A JUNK-FOOD WORLD

[1]Maureen Salaman and James F. Scheer, Foods That Heal, (Menlo Park, CA: Statford Publishing Inc., 1989), p. 102.
[2]Ibid.
[3]Ibid., pp. 102,103.
[4]Ibid., p. 103.
[5]Ibid., pp. 103,104.
[6]Ibid., p. 104.
[7]Ibid., p. 105.
[8]Ibid., pp. 105,106.
[9]Jeffrey R.M. Kunz, MD and Asher J. Finkel, MD eds., The American Medical Association Family Medical Guide, (New York: Random House, Inc., 1987), pp. 663,664.
[10]Ibid., pp. 664,665.
[11]Ibid., p. 664.
[12]Salaman (Foods That Heal), op. cit., p. 104.
[13]Ibid.
[14]Kunz, op. cit., p. 664.
[15]Ibid.
[16]Ibid.
[17]Ibid.
[18]Ibid., p. 529.
[19]Salaman (Foods That Heal), op. cit., pp. 84-86.
[20]Ibid., pp. 312-317.
[21]Kunz., op. cit., pp. 725,726.

[22]Ibid.

[23]Salaman (Foods That Heal), op. cit., pp. 12-14.

[24]Kunz., op. cit., pp. 730,731.

[25]Salaman (Foods That Heal), op. cit., pp. 16-20.

[26]Maureen Salaman, Foods That Heal, Cravings/Addictions, Conquer Cravings For: Chocolate, Alcohol & Tobacco!, (Menlo Park, CA: Maureen Salaman's Nutritional Ministries).

[27]Salaman (Foods That Heal), op. cit., pp. 270-275.

[28]Ibid., pp. 37-42.

[29]Ibid., pp. 394-396.

[30]Ibid., pp. 98-100.

[31]Ibid., pp. 158-160.

SECTION 8
NUTRITION VS. THE AGING PROCESS

[1]Maureen Salaman, The Diet Bible: The Bible For Dieters, (Menlo Park, CA: Statford Publishing Inc., 1990), pp. 105,106.

[2]Jeffrey R.M. Kunz, MD and Asher J. Finkel, MD, eds., The American Medical Association Family Medical Guide, (New York: Random House, Inc., 1987), p. 529.

[3]Maureen Salaman and James F. Scheer, Foods That Heal, (Menlo Park, CA: Statford Publishing Inc., 1989), pp. 212-218.

[4]Salaman (Foods That Heal), op. cit., pp. 458-461.

[5]Ibid., pp. 479-485.

[6]"Has Growing Older Placed you at Nutritional Risk?" Tufts University Diet and Nutrition Letter [New York], May 1992, p. 3.

[7]Ibid.

[8]Ibid., pp. 4,5.

[9]Ibid., p. 4.

[10]Salaman (Foods That Heal), op. cit., pp. 51-53.

[11]Tufts University Diet and Nutrition Letter, op. cit., p. 4.

[12]Kunz, op. cit., pp. 496,497.

[13]Salaman (Foods That Heal), op. cit., pp. 16-20.

[14]Ibid., pp. 355-357.

[15]Ibid., pp. 28-34.
[16]Ibid., pp. 55-63.
[17]Ibid., pp. 123-126.
[18]Ibid., pp. 162,163.
[19]Ibid., pp. 175-179.
[20]Ibid., pp. 171-174.
[21]Ibid., pp. 192-196.
[22]Ibid., pp. 319-326.
[23]Ibid., pp. 380-384.
[24]Ibid., pp. 385-391.

SECTION 10
RECIPES FOR HEALTHY LIVING

[1]Brian Edmonds, The Doctor's Book of Bible Healing Foods, (Boca Raton, FL: Globe Communications Corp., 1992), pp. 19,20.

WORKS CITED

"Defining Major Depression." Rocky Mountain News [Denver, CO] 12 April 1993: sec. A: 24.

Diamond, Harvey, and Marilyn Diamond. Fit For Life II: Living Health. New York: Warner Books, Inc., 1987.

Edmonds, Brian. The Doctor's Book of Bible Healing Foods. Boca Raton, FL: Globe Communications Corp., 1992.

Finkel, Asher J. MD and Jeffrey R.M. Kunz, MD, eds. The American Medical Association Family Medical Guide. New York: Random House, Inc., 1987.

"Has Growing Older Placed You at Nutritional Risk?" Tufts University Diet and Nutrition Letter. New York: May 1992: 3.

Kloss, Jethro. Back to Eden. New York: Lancer Books, Inc., 1971.

Mycoskie, Pam. Butter Busters The Cookbook. Arlington, TX: Butter Busters Publishing, 1992.

O'Brien, James. Super Foods. Boca Raton, FL: Globe Communications Corp., 1992.

Omartian, Stormie. Greater Health—God's Way: Seven Steps to Health, Youthfulness and Vitality. Chatsworth, CA: Sparrow Press, 1984.

_____. A Step in the Right Direction: Your Guide to Inner Happiness. Nashville: Thomas Nelson Publishers, 1984.

Salaman, Maureen. Foods That Heal, Cravings/Addictions, Conquer Cravings For: Chocolate, Alcohol & Tobacco! Menlo Park, CA: Maureen Salaman's Nutritional Ministries.

_____. Nutrition: The Cancer Answer. Menlo Park, CA: Statford Publishing Inc., 1984.

_____. The Diet Bible: The Bible For Dieters. Menlo Park, CA: Statford Publishing Inc., 1990.

Salaman, Maureen and James F. Scheer. Foods That Heal. Menlo Park, CA: Statford Publishing Inc., 1989.

Sheehy, Gail. The Silent Passage Menopause. New York: Random House, Inc., 1991.

Stevens, Susan, M.A., R.D. Delitefully HealthMark . . . Cooking for the Health of It! Lakewood, CO: SWS Publishing, 1989.

"Study Puts Doctors on Alert for Patients Suffering Depression." Rocky Mountain News [Denver, CO] 12 April, 1993: sec. A: 2.

Tarkan, Laurie. "5 Moves That Trim It All." Family Circle [New York] 23 February 1993: 82,83.

Wade, Carlson. The Miracle of Bible Healing Foods. Boca Raton, FL: Globe Communications Corp., 1991.

Receive Jesus Christ as Lord and Savior of Your Life.

The Bible says, *"That if thou shalt confess with thy mouth the Lord Jesus, and shalt believe in thine heart that God raised him from the dead, thou shalt be saved. For with the heart man believeth unto righteousness; and with the mouth confession is made unto salvation"* (Romans 10:9,10).

To receive Jesus Christ as Lord and Savior of your life, sincerely pray this prayer from your heart:

Dear Jesus,

I believe that You died for me and that You rose again on the third day. I confess to You that I am a sinner and that I need Your love and forgiveness. Come into my life, forgive my sins, and give me eternal life. I confess You now as my Lord. Thank You for my salvation!

Signed _____ Date _____

Mr. & Mrs.
Mr.
Name Miss _____ Please print.
Mrs.

Address _____

City _____ State ____ Zip _____

Phone (H)( ) _____

Write to us.
We will send you information to help you
with your new life in Christ.

Marilyn Hickey Ministries
P.O. Box 17340 • Denver, CO 80217 • 303-770-0400
www.mhmin.org

For Your Information
Free Monthly Magazine

☐ Please send me your free monthly magazine
OUTPOURING (including daily devotionals,
timely articles, and ministry updates)!

Tapes and Books

☐ Please send me Marilyn's latest product catalog.

Please print.

Mr. & Mrs.
Miss
Mrs.
Name Mr. _____

Address _____

City _____

State _____ Zip _____

Phone (H) ( ) _____

(W) ( ) _____

Mail to
Marilyn Hickey Ministries
P.O. Box 17340
Denver, CO 80217
(303) 770-0400

Prayer Request(s)

Let us join our faith with yours for your prayer needs. Fill out the coupon below and send to Marilyn Hickey Ministries, P.O. Box 17340, Denver, CO 80217.

Prayer Request(s) _____

_____

_____

_____

_____

_____

Mr. & Mrs.   Please print.
Mr.
Name Miss_____
Mrs.

Address _____

City _____

State _____ Zip _____

Phone(H) (   ) _____

(W) (   ) _____

If you want prayer immediately, call our Prayer Center
at 303-796-1333, Monday—Friday,
4 a.m.—4:30 p.m. (MT).

BOOKS BY MARILYN HICKEY

A Cry for Miracles $7.95
Acts of the Holy Spirit $7.95
Angels All Around $7.95
Armageddon $4.95
Ask Marilyn $9.95
Be Healed $9.95
Bible Encounter Classic Edition $24.95
Blessing Journal $4.95
Book of Revelation Comic Book (The) $3.00
Break the Generation Curse $7.95
Break the Generation Curse –Part 2 .... $9.95
Building Blocks for Better Families $4.95
Daily Devotional $7.95
Dear Marilyn $7.95
Devils, Demons, and Deliverance $9.95
Divorce Is Not the Answer $7.95
Especially for Today's Woman $14.95
Freedom From Bondages $7.95
Gift-Wrapped Fruit $2.95
God's Covenant for Your Family $7.95
God's Rx for a Hurting Heart $4.95
Hebrew Honey $14.95
How to Be a Mature Christian $7.95
Know Your Ministry $4.95
Maximize Your Day . . . God's Way $7.95
Miracle Signs and Wonders $24.95
Names of God (The) $7.95
Nehemiah—Rebuilding the Broken Places in Your Life $7.95
No. 1 Key to Success—Meditation (The) $4.95
Proverbs Classic Library Edition $24.95
Release the Power of the Blood Covenant $4.95
Satan-Proof Your Home $7.95
Save the Family Promise Book $14.95
Signs in the Heavens $7.95
What Every Person Wants to Know About Prayer $4.95
When Only a Miracle Will Do $4.95
Your Miracle Source $4.95
Your Total Health Handbook—Body • Soul • Spirit $9.95

Marilyn Hickey Ministries

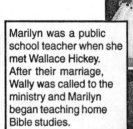

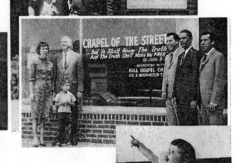

Marilyn was a public school teacher when she met Wallace Hickey. After their marriage, Wally was called to the ministry and Marilyn began teaching home Bible studies.

The vision of Marilyn Hickey Ministries is to "cover the earth with the Word" (Isaiah 11:9). For over 30 years Marilyn Hickey has dedicated herself to an anointed, unique, and distinguished ministry of reaching out to people—from all walks of life—who are hungry for God's Word and all that He has for them. Millions have witnessed and acclaimed the positive, personal impact she brings through fresh revelation knowledge that God has given her through His Word.

Marilyn has been the invited guest of government leaders and heads of state from many nations of the world. She is considered by many to be one of today's greatest ambassadors of God's Good News to this dark and hurting generation.

The more Marilyn follows God's will for her life, the more God uses her to bring refreshing, renewal, and revival to the Body of Christ throughout the world. As His obedient servant, Marilyn desires to follow Him all the days of her life.

Marilyn and Wally adopted their son Michael; through a fulfilled prophecy they had their daughter Sarah, who with her husband Reece, is now part of the ministry.

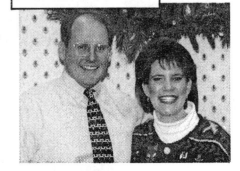

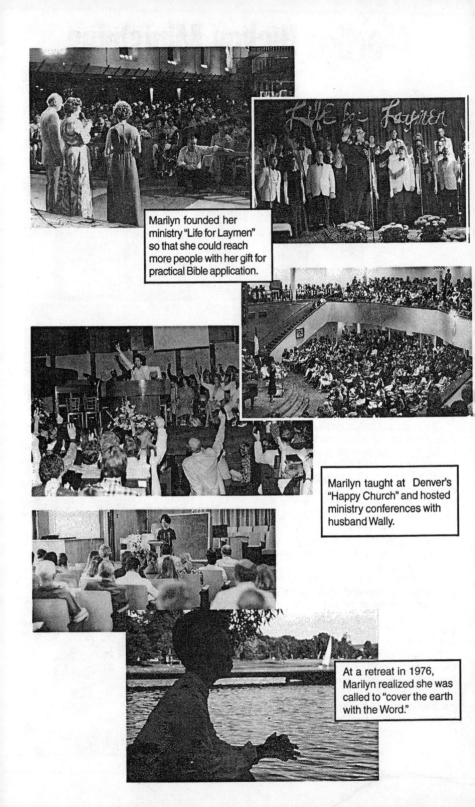

Marilyn founded her ministry "Life for Laymen" so that she could reach more people with her gift for practical Bible application.

Marilyn taught at Denver's "Happy Church" and hosted ministry conferences with husband Wally.

At a retreat in 1976, Marilyn realized she was called to "cover the earth with the Word."

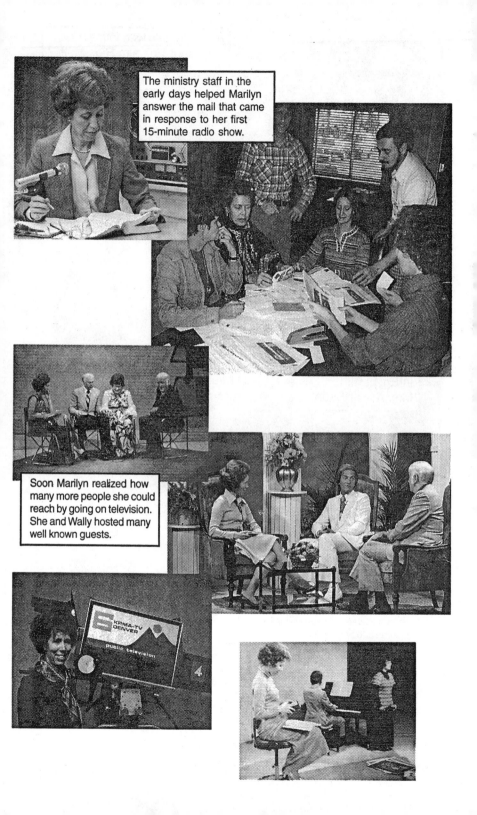

The ministry staff in the early days helped Marilyn answer the mail that came in response to her first 15-minute radio show.

Soon Marilyn realized how many more people she could reach by going on television. She and Wally hosted many well known guests.

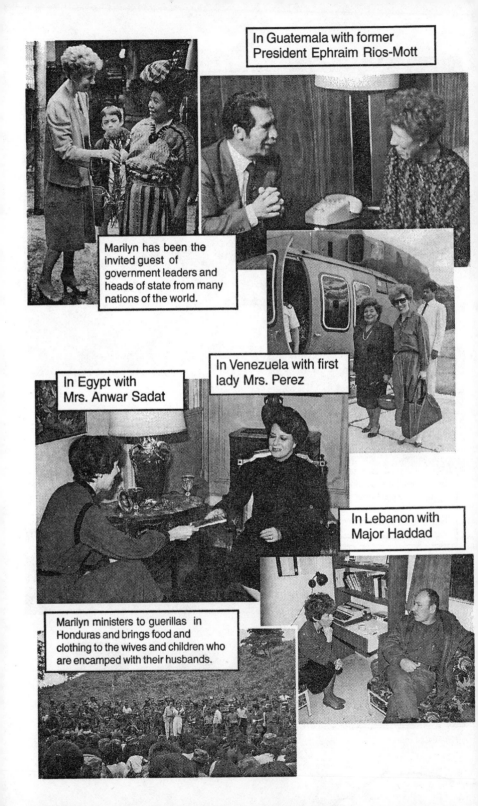

In Guatemala with former President Ephraim Rios-Mott

Marilyn has been the invited guest of government leaders and heads of state from many nations of the world.

In Egypt with Mrs. Anwar Sadat

In Venezuela with first lady Mrs. Perez

In Lebanon with Major Haddad

Marilyn ministers to guerillas in Honduras and brings food and clothing to the wives and children who are encamped with their husbands.

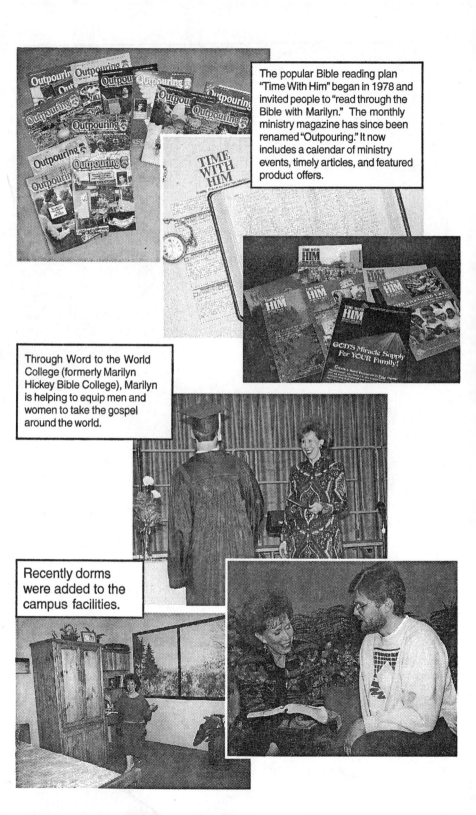

The popular Bible reading plan "Time With Him" began in 1978 and invited people to "read through the Bible with Marilyn." The monthly ministry magazine has since been renamed "Outpouring." It now includes a calendar of ministry events, timely articles, and featured product offers.

Through Word to the World College (formerly Marilyn Hickey Bible College), Marilyn is helping to equip men and women to take the gospel around the world.

Recently dorms were added to the campus facilities.

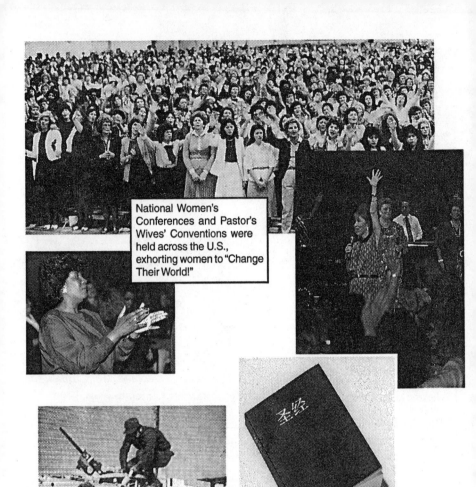

National Women's Conferences and Pastor's Wives' Conventions were held across the U.S., exhorting women to "Change Their World!"

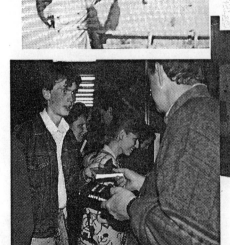

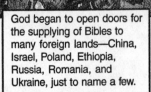

God began to open doors for the supplying of Bibles to many foreign lands—China, Israel, Poland, Ethiopia, Russia, Romania, and Ukraine, just to name a few.

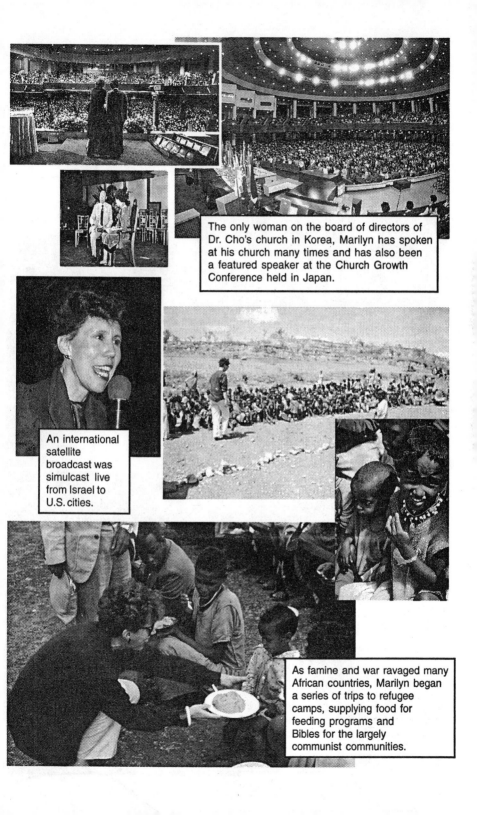

The only woman on the board of directors of Dr. Cho's church in Korea, Marilyn has spoken at his church many times and has also been a featured speaker at the Church Growth Conference held in Japan.

An international satellite broadcast was simulcast live from Israel to U.S. cities.

As famine and war ravaged many African countries, Marilyn began a series of trips to refugee camps, supplying food for feeding programs and Bibles for the largely communist communities.

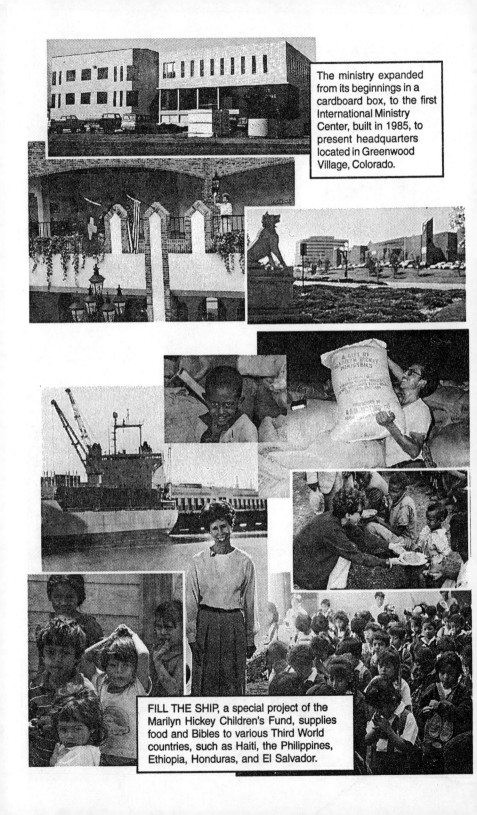

The ministry expanded from its beginnings in a cardboard box, to the first International Ministry Center, built in 1985, to present headquarters located in Greenwood Village, Colorado.

FILL THE SHIP, a special project of the Marilyn Hickey Children's Fund, supplies food and Bibles to various Third World countries, such as Haiti, the Philippines, Ethiopia, Honduras, and El Salvador.

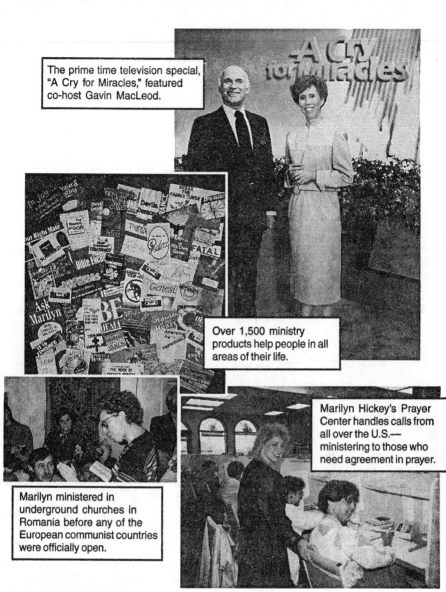

The prime time television special, "A Cry for Miracles," featured co-host Gavin MacLeod.

Over 1,500 ministry products help people in all areas of their life.

Marilyn Hickey's Prayer Center handles calls from all over the U.S.— ministering to those who need agreement in prayer.

Marilyn ministered in underground churches in Romania before any of the European communist countries were officially open.

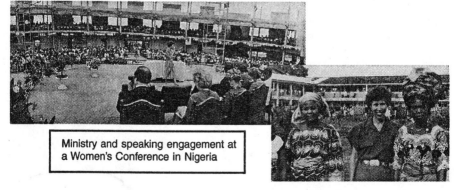

Ministry and speaking engagement at a Women's Conference in Nigeria

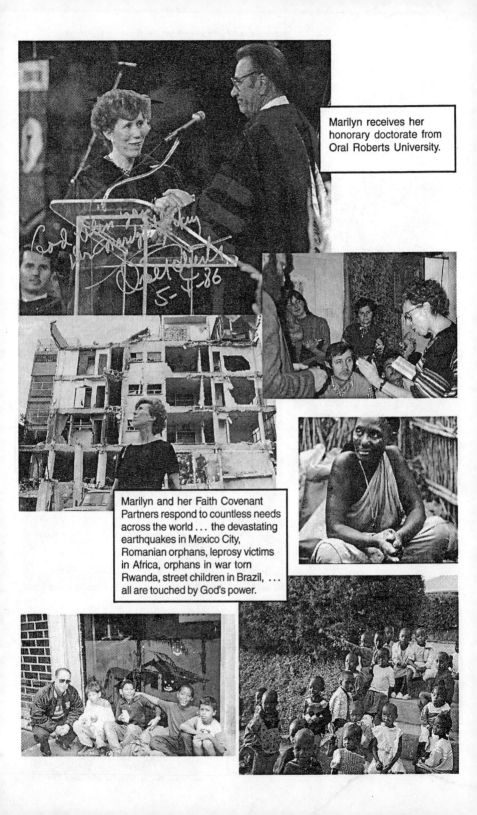

Marilyn receives her honorary doctorate from Oral Roberts University.

Marilyn and her Faith Covenant Partners respond to countless needs across the world ... the devastating earthquakes in Mexico City, Romanian orphans, leprosy victims in Africa, orphans in war torn Rwanda, street children in Brazil, ... all are touched by God's power.

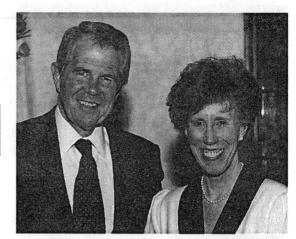

Marilyn has been a guest several times on the 700 Club with host Pat Robertson.

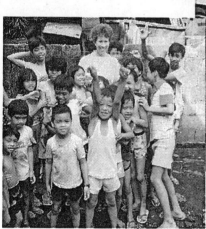

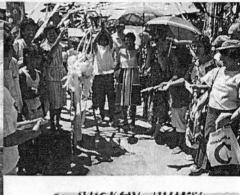

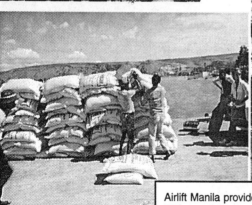

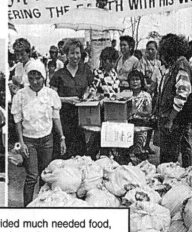

Airlift Manila provided much needed food, Bibles, and personal supplies to the Philippines; MHM also raised funds to aid in the digging of water wells for those without clean drinking water.

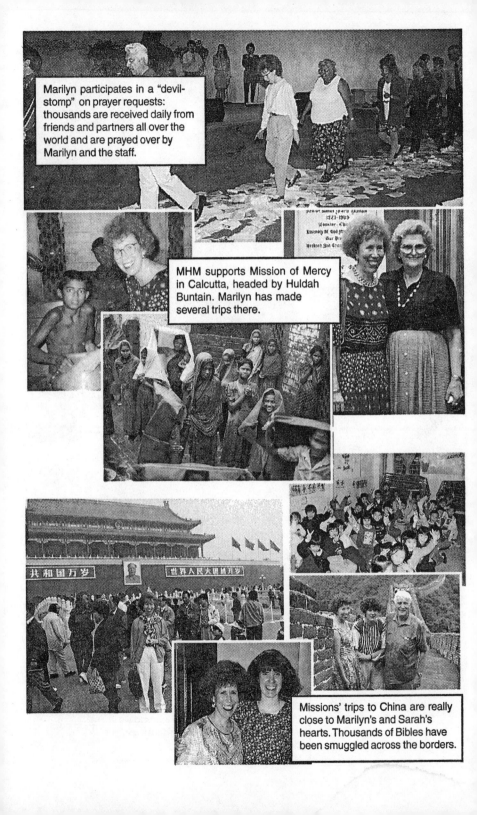

Marilyn participates in a "devil-stomp" on prayer requests: thousands are received daily from friends and partners all over the world and are prayed over by Marilyn and the staff.

MHM supports Mission of Mercy in Calcutta, headed by Huldah Buntain. Marilyn has made several trips there.

Missions' trips to China are really close to Marilyn's and Sarah's hearts. Thousands of Bibles have been smuggled across the borders.

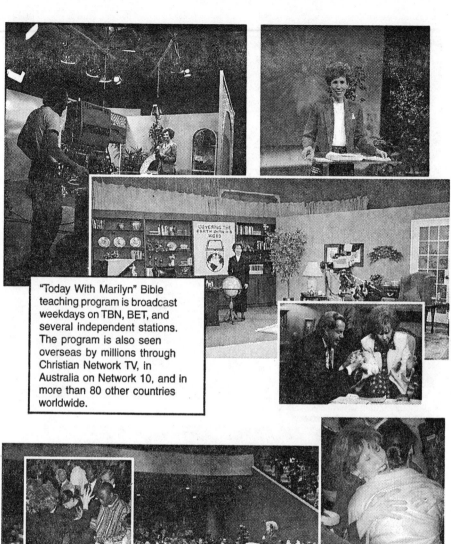

"Today With Marilyn" Bible teaching program is broadcast weekdays on TBN, BET, and several independent stations. The program is also seen overseas by millions through Christian Network TV, in Australia on Network 10, and in more than 80 other countries worldwide.

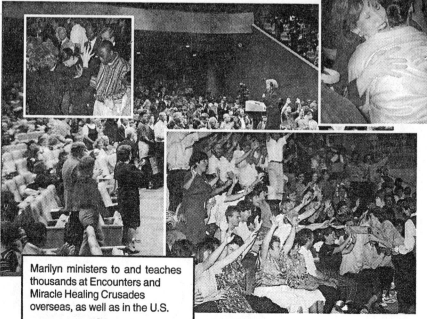

Marilyn ministers to and teaches thousands at Encounters and Miracle Healing Crusades overseas, as well as in the U.S.

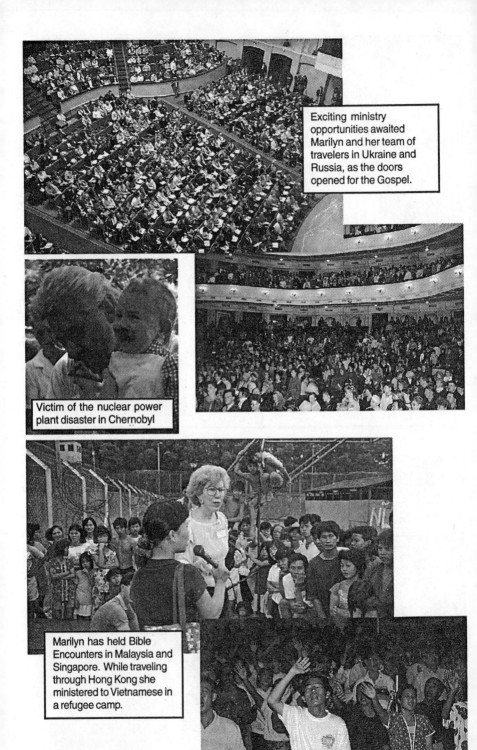

Exciting ministry opportunities awaited Marilyn and her team of travelers in Ukraine and Russia, as the doors opened for the Gospel.

Victim of the nuclear power plant disaster in Chernobyl

Marilyn has held Bible Encounters in Malaysia and Singapore. While traveling through Hong Kong she ministered to Vietnamese in a refugee camp.

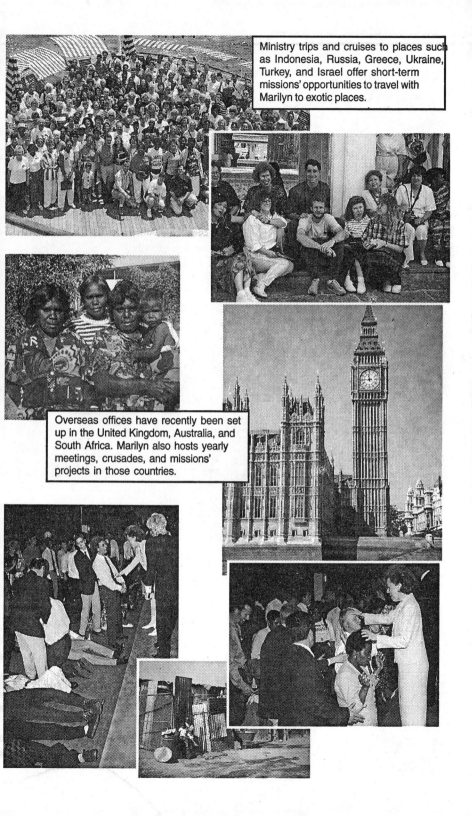

Ministry trips and cruises to places such as Indonesia, Russia, Greece, Ukraine, Turkey, and Israel offer short-term missions' opportunities to travel with Marilyn to exotic places.

Overseas offices have recently been set up in the United Kingdom, Australia, and South Africa. Marilyn also hosts yearly meetings, crusades, and missions' projects in those countries.

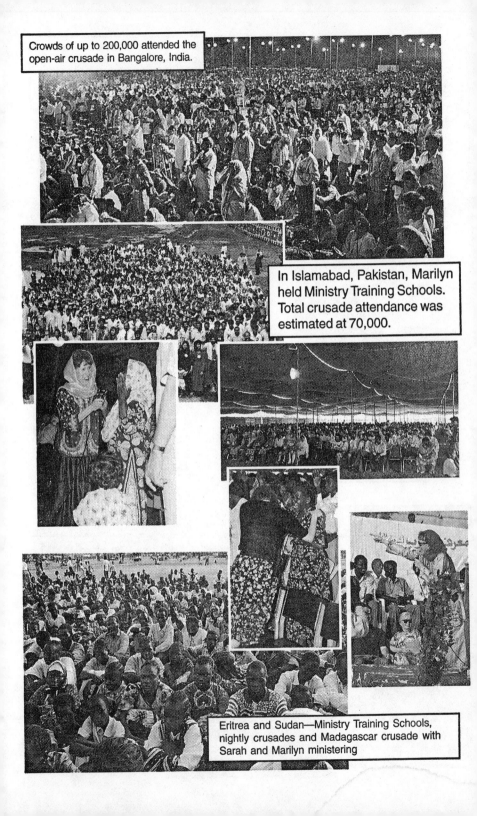

Crowds of up to 200,000 attended the open-air crusade in Bangalore, India.

In Islamabad, Pakistan, Marilyn held Ministry Training Schools. Total crusade attendance was estimated at 70,000.

Eritrea and Sudan—Ministry Training Schools, nightly crusades and Madagascar crusade with Sarah and Marilyn ministering